30/12

GW00546912

Diary
A Hair Transplant

A Journalist's Search For David Cassidy Hair

By Brian Beacon

Regards, and great to meet you,

Brian -

PHANTOM
PUBLISHING UK

Copyright © Brian Beacom

First published in the UK in 2008 by Phantom Publishing
UK, 82 Mitchell Street, Glasgow, G1 3NA

All rights reserved. No part of this publication may be
reproduced, stored in a retrieval system, or transmitted
in any form or by any means, electronic, mechanical,
photo-copying, recording or otherwise, without the prior
permission in writing of the publishers.

ISBN: 978-0-9561322-0-8

Printing by Norhaven A/S
Edited by Brenda Paterson.

Thanks to Mick at Farjo.

PHANTOM
PUBLISHING UK

Brian Beacom is the Showbiz Editor of the Evening Times in Glasgow.

He has written two celebrity biographies and is currently working on a biography of Stanley Baxter and a book of (allegedly) hilarious theatre stories.

He lives in the Renfrewshire village of Kilmacolm with two cats, Effie and Simba, who were dumped upon him when his partner moved in.

This book is dedicated to Christopher Beacom.

Contents

Part 2

1
Peek-a-boo Hair

APRIL 30, 2008. HT Day. Hair Transplant Day.
It's 7.15am. I'm on a train to Manchester, staring out of
the window and into the past.

I love this city. It reminds me of university days and
going to the football with my pal Brendan from Stretford.
More poignantly, it reminds me of an ex called Julie who
had wavy blond peek-a-boo hair and looked like a Forties
film star.

Ah, Julie. It's no surprise she finds herself cut and
pasted back onto the memory page at this very moment.
She once predicted, (showing a rare sign of insensitivity)
that my David Cassidy-like locks would be gone by my late
twenties. I was 22 at the time and this was not what I
wanted to hear at all. Bald? I couldn't bear the thought
of it. Baldness, after all, had a negative association.

I wanted to become a journalist since I was a kid and
discovered that Superman's alter ego Clark Kent was a
reporter. But at the same time I learned his arch enemy
and world destroyer Lex Luthor was bald. And I realised
that bald guys in comics were almost always the bad guys.
And movies of course.James Bond wore a wig, because

good guys always have hair, but Odd-Job and Blofeld were egg-heads.

Cartoons also depicted bald people as being baddies. Little Elmer Fudd was bald, a shotgun-armed psychopath who spent his life trying to blow Bugs Bunny's brains out.

But most importantly, in fiction and in life, bald guys never, ever, got the girls. Was I set to lose out on the wavy-haired Julies of this world?

The flashback is halted by the halting of the train. Now, I'm stepping off and into a bright, vibrant Piccadilly Station. And I feel wonderful. And anxious. Why this oxymoronic state? Well, I'm about to undergo hair transplant surgery that will give me a covering on my head that I haven't had for years.

Today is the day I get new hair. Well, not new hair. It's old hair actually, but it will be moved – like Pickfords, but with follicles - from the back of my head to a new home on my scalp.

Yet, at the same time I'm trepidatious. Not so much at the idea of surgery, the thought of pain or the sight of swelling, because I have real faith in the doctor carrying out the procedure. But because I'm not entirely convinced that it will all work out as it's supposed to. I've done all my research, and I feel I've made the right choice of transplant surgeon. However, I've also spent years reading about the hair transplants that have gone horribly wrong.

Or even just not quite turned out right.

Will my new hair grow in the right direction? Will the hairline look natural? What if, after thirty years of dreaming about having new hair, the results turn out to be a nightmare and I'm left with nothing?

I don't get the chance to dwell on this thought because the train has stopped and I'm off and walking towards the barrier.

On the other side is Mick, the hair clinic's manager. And I'm glad he's met me because he's a no-nonsense, likeable bloke in his forties with a reassuring smile.

"How did you sleep," he says, enquiring of my hotel stay the night before. Unfortunately I'd chosen to come down to Manchester on a day United were playing Barcelona and there was more chance of me getting a game for them than finding a hotel room in the city.

As a result, I'd had to opt for a hotel in Crewe, conveniently, next to the train station.

"I slept well," I said. "The gentle thunder of the trains that ran right underneath the hotel had a strangely soporific effect. In fact, I must sleep directly above 300 wt of moving diesel more often."

He laughed and so did I. We both knew it was good to get the day off on a smile. But I was still unsure. What if we get to the clinic and the old hair won't want to be repositioned? What if Dr Farjo, the man whose hands my head will soon be placed in, discovers a problem and decides my skull isn't suitable for shifting hair around on after all?

Yes, my hair has been falling out for the longest time. I've known for some time I would be a statistic, one of the forty per cent of men who suffer from male pattern baldness by the age of thirty-five. And I'm determined to halt the hair loss process. But will the result be as exciting as the last few months of expectation?

'Of course it will,' I tell myself.

As we step into the Manchester sunshine I look for a sign. Any sign that will convince me this will all work out

3

in the end. And just as we make our way in the direction of Chorlton Street, a tram passes. And on the tram is a giant shampoo ad.

'That'll do,' I think, smiling.

Two minutes later and we are in the lift in a very swish building making our way up to the Sixth Floor. Inside, the clock in the reception area reveals it's just 7.30am, but already the place is a hive of industry. Mick leaves me in reception to wait a few moments until he has a chat with Dr Farjo.

I had been in the Farjo Clinic before, for the initial consultation five months ago. But because of all the excitement going on in my head I realised I hadn't picked up on detail; a bit like viewing a house for the first time. This time around my eye catches the *Before* and *After* pics on the wall. And I realise one of the blokes looks familiar. He should. It's Mick. Ten years ago, I later discover, Mick had hair like mine is today; thin and patchy and not long for the world that is the top of my head. But today Mick has hair. A pretty good head of hair at that. I take this as Another Sign. A really good sign.

"Dr Farjo will see you now," calls out Mick, who is walking into the reception area.

And I move through the corridors, into Bessam Farjo's office where I'm alone for a couple of minutes. Again, I get to take in the view of the walls. And this time around I see they are covered in framed certificates, with memberships of world-wide hair transplant organisations, with details of conferences and seminars attended. Dr Farjo has a list of accreditations that are as long as Rapunzel's hair. It's obvious this is a man who knows hair replacement.

This is Another Good Sign.

"Hi, how are you?" says the cheery Iraq-born doctor who will relocate my hair to a far happier place. And now we're chatting, about my trip down from Glasgow, about Manchester United's win. And about the upcoming procedure. And he's telling me how straight-forward it will all be.

Now, some doctors don't instil confidence. I remember once going to hospital with a knee problem and being addressed by a young locum who wore ankle-height cream trainers, a grubby t-shirt and spoke to me through a runny nose which he wiped episodically with the sleeve of his tatty white coat. He told me I had Housewife's Knee. But because of his appalling presentation I wouldn't have believed him if he produced an actual eighty year-old for comparison purposes.

Dr Farjo however has a reassuring manner.

"Take these pills," he says, offering a clutch of small blue tablets which he says are anti-infection agents, and one white one.

"The Valium is to make you really feel relaxed."

Half an hour later I most certainly am. And I'm in the clinic relaxing in a large leather reclining chair, the sort British Airways charge three grand for on a First Class long haul flight. I'm laying back facing a big plasma screen and listening to the laid-back Terry Wogan on the radio. Considering what's about to happen to me, and the importance of it all, I'm amazingly laid-back.

'This is way, way better than a day in a busy newspaper office,' I say to myself. And so far, it's true.

Dr Farjo re-covers what he explained before in my consultation meeting about what the procedure would involve. During the course of the day a strip will be removed from the back of my head, dissected into follicular units – groups of hairs - and those units inserted into my scalp.

And this process will carry on most of the day, but there will be a break for lunch, and I can order up a sandwich and drink. It all sounds fine. I'm then told there are a selection of recent movies to watch or, for the moment, I can listen to Terry Wogan on the radio. Ah, Tel. The gentle voice that introduces gentle music to genteel people. And I listen and become even more relaxed.

Meanwhile, Dr Farjo is kneading my head, moving my scalp around with his fingers, like he were making bread.

"Yes, there's good movement here," he says. "You have good scalp laxity."

"Great!" I say, enthusiastically, without really knowing why. I suppose if he's happy . . . Later however the significance of having an elastic scalp will become very obvious to me.

Then Dr Farjo puts a band around my head. I imagine it's something to do with restricting blood supply during the procedure but I don't ask, probably because of the Valium. And he announces he's about to shave off what's left of the hair on top of my head, the 20 or 30 remaining hairs that have been carefully re-arranged so's to look like 35 or 40. Panic time.

"Eh? Shave my head? Not in a million years! Turn me into Kojak? You can't. In fact, I'll look worse than Kojak because I'll have hair at the sides. I'll look like Max Wall's younger brother or that odd-ball Keith Flint from the Prodigy.

"I didn't know about having my head shaved. I thought the transplanted hair would be happily introduced to the existing filaments and they'd get on famously and live happily ever after. Or at least until the old hair fell out in it's own good time.

"I'm out of here!"

'The best thing to do is to
behave in a manner befitting one's age. If you
are sixteen and under, try not to go bald.'

~ Woody Allen.

2
Numbskull

I DON'T say any of this to Dr F of course. I just think it. But I'm still hugely reluctant to have a totally bald, shiny head – the image of my own personal hell. Part of my brain however remembers that Dr Farjo told me he needs a cleared landscape to see where he's planting - and I keep quiet – while swallowing a little lump in my throat.

If it weren't for the relaxant, I'd probably have dropped a couple of tears at the realisation I was about to have a completely bald dome for the first time in my life.

Bzzzzzz. He's shaving away my last remaining scalp hair. I'm saying goodbye to old friends. But I console myself with the thought I'll see them again in about two months when they (hopefully) grow back in. Now, Dr Farjo is pulling out his marker pen. He's drawing lines on my head, the outlines for the new hairlines as he did during the consultation.

He lifts a mirror and shows me how the final result will look. But I'm not excited. In fact, I'm not sure at all, but not because it doesn't look as though I'll have much hair at the front. The opposite. I think he's giving me too much of a hairline and it won't look entirely realistic.

I'll look like Scott Tracy from Thunderbirds.

"Are you sure it's not too hopeful?" I ask.

"No, it will look great," he says.

Now, I almost feel like debating the issue. Debate is all too often the default position I take up. But I don't.

'Trust the process,' I tell myself. 'Relax.'

And I do. And it's not so hard because Terry is playing Newton Faulkner's new single and it's great. And my mind starts to wander in the direction of Wogan himself. And I'm now happy because if it weren't for this process I could be wearing a wig. Like Terry. As sure as Limerick summer rain, the radio icon wears hair that does not grow naturally from his head. He has done so since the days when the *Eurovision Song Contest* was fair. I had this information 30 years ago on good authority, gained when I went along to one of these high street hair treatment centres.

Now, ostensibly I didn't go because of my own hair problem; I still had David Cassidy hair at the time. I was riding shotgun on the trip with my pal, Sparky. Sparky, at just 17, was waking up every morning to find clumps of his hair laying cold and dead on his pillow. After trying to come to terms with it for a few years, and failing, he was seduced by this treatment centre in Glasgow; you know the sort, one of these places that offers '*A Whole New Look*.' And it made claims such as '*We Can Halt Your Hair Loss*,' and '*Hair Loss Can Be A Thing Of The Past*.'

What they really could do, very well, I discovered, was convince fragile young men like Sparky – and Wogan perhaps - that the way to 'cure' baldness was by pretending to have real hair. No sooner were we in the door than

Sparky had a sample wig slapped to his head - and combed in a modern style faster than you can say 'Made in Korea From Real Human Hair.'

"Terry Wogan wears one just like this," said the salesman/consultant.

And, to be honest, the Terrywig did look quite good. And Sparky - bold, bare soul that he was - ordered one of these custom-made rugs. And to be even more honest, when it was fitted a few weeks later most people didn't know it wasn't home-grown. Sparky and me went off to uni shortly afterwards (we were late starters) and he had the confidence to get the girls.

But while Sparky was going through with the business of wig-fitting I wasn't simply playing the role of Supportive Friend. You see, I already had my own hair worries. What Veronica Lake look-alike Julie didn't know was that she *wasn't* educating me to the probability of my own hair loss. I was already aware. Frighteningly aware.

On August 22nd 1974, – the day after I left home – I washed my 18 year-old head in a crotchety Hull landlady's sink and as I pulled out the plug and watched the water swirl around the vortex I realised it was disappearing a little more slowly than it should. The reason? The plug hole was blocked. By some of my David Cassidy hair.

On realisation, my heart stopped for an instant. "Oh flip!" I howled. (Not the actual word used).

The next day I did some research and learned that most men see around 25-100 strands a day go down the plughole. (Until this point I hadn't seen any leave my head; battleaxe landlady stress-induced?)

But nor was I comforted by the stats which revealed that around two-thirds of men are either bald or close to checking into the Follicle Free Hotel by the age of 60.

That's why when Sparky went along to the hair treatment centre, part of me was there to watch and learn. Was wig wearing – like Sparky and Terry – to be my future?

"Now, I've shaved the donor area and I'm now removing the strip containing your hair follicles," says Dr Farjo, cutting into my thoughts and the back of my head.

"Fantastic!" I say. And I'm genuinely delighted at the very thought of it.

We're progressing. We're moving ahead. On my head. This thin strip of scalp, about half an inch wide and running from above each ear and around my head contains the hair roots which are 'genetically programmed to grow for the rest of your life', ie. the area where men rarely go bald.

Once Dr Farjo has removed the strip, he tells me he will then use stereoscopic dissecting microscopes to divide this donor area into the individual follicular unit grafts.

Hairs don't, for the most part, grow in isolation. They grow in units. Follicular Units, he had explained to me earlier are the natural groupings of the hairs in their original habitat. These units contain between 1-4 hairs with the average being 2.2.

Modern-day hair transplantation is all about keeping these FUs intact when transferring them to the top of the head site. This results in better survival of the hairs - and a more natural-looking result. But of course, it means much more work for a surgeon, and takes much more time.

"Can you feel anything?" asks Dr Farjo.

Well, I can. I can feel him slice into the outer layer of the back of my head. It isn't painful however. The head has been anaesthetized so the worst I'm feeling is slight discomfort. And after a few minutes the hair strip has been removed.

"I'm going to start stitching you up now," says Dr Farjo.

"Great, go for it," I say, smiling now, as if he had just told me he was getting me a juice from the fridge.

But at least I'm relaxed again. And my mind wanders back in the direction of Sparky. During our time at university I realised his wig-wearing life was not for me. Sparky revealed how he taped his wig onto his head every day - and it all seemed so demanding.

And I came to realise on some days that his nice piece didn't always sit nicely at the nape of his neck. He told me in fact he had to have two wigs, so that one could be treated and repaired while he wore the other. But there was no other option. Sparky was just like Sinatra, John Wayne and Charlton Heston. They didn't want the world to know they were bald. (At least film stars had personal hairdressers who made sure the wigs – on screen at least – were almost undetectable.)

Oddly enough, a couple of years after leaving university, in the early Eighties, I had my own personal hairdresser. And he couldn't convince me wigs were an option.

I landed a job writing for an entertainment agency in Toronto, and lived with my little hairdresser uncle Chris - who wore a hairpiece for most of his adult life. (He maintained that being a bald teasy weasy was never an option).

Now, my dad wasn't bald, he had thick, dark, Clark Gable hair (and also most of his vices) but my grandfather's genetic barricades against baldness hadn't been passed down the line to me, or to Chris. Chris however had a relaxed attitude to hair loss. Off duty. Then in his mid-fifties and still playing football, just before running onto the pitch for his Toronto Sunday league matches he'd yank off his wig in front of his soccer buddies and throw it on top of the beer cooler. But he didn't want clients to know he wore a wig. He wanted to appear as he did in the black and white portrait pic on his salon wall of him in his younger days, in which he wore a Peter Lawford hairstyle, a sharp dark suit, a thin black tie and a slightly devilish grin.

During the last 20 years of his life he looked for a baldness cure. Not for himself; he reckoned he was beyond hope, but for young people, like his favourite nephew, who would be spared the ignominy of taping fake hair to their head.

While giving me the regular freebie, he'd noticed my locks were becoming less Cassidy-thick and knew things would only get worse if left to Mother Nature. So he'd come out with all sorts of lotions and potions for me to try. And I tried them. I rubbed this snake oil or whatever it was made up of it into my scalp every day for months but the only thing it restored was hair product company profits.

Meanwhile, living with a wig-wearing hairdresser was an education. I learned to spot a piece at 50 yards. (I've never figured out why so many men in their sixties or older wear wigs with more hair than Tarzan? Why not have just the right amount, go for verisimilitude?)

But what I certainly learned was that I never, ever wanted to wear one. No. Not me. These taped-on hair pieces offered little more than brief illusion of attractiveness, the hair covering equivalent of Meg Ryan; appear on Parkinson's chat show for a couple of minutes and the reality is soon discovered.

Sparky too came to that conclusion because after a couple of years his own wig-wearing days were knocked on the head.

He gave up on his new hair because the fear of discovery and revelation (at what point when you go out with a girl do you admit you are wearing someone else's hair on your head?) became greater than the fear of being called 'Baldy.

Chris however, was always a source of hope to me. He followed the progress of the Canadian hair treatment centres with a Mountie-like dogged determination.

And one day he reported that there would be a solution. Hair transplants will solve all the problems of the world's bald men," announced my uncle the Hair Prophet.

"Thank goodness," I thought.

And now here I am in the process of having one.

'Hollywood is no place to be bald in.'

~ **Time Magazine**

3

Elton's Squares

IT'S now around 10am and I know this because Wogan has switched off for the day. It's Ken Bruce's turn at the microphone and he's a nice presenter, but it grates with me a little that Irishman Terry broadcasts in the guise of Home Counties faux pompous oaf - and then Scotsman Ken appears and plays the same character.

However Dr Farjo, who's perhaps even more sensitive than I had imagined, picks up on my Bruce-induced distress which the Valium has clearly failed to quell.

"Would you like to watch a movie?" he asks as he implants Follicular Units containing single hair into the front of my head, creating my new hairline.

"We've got quite a selection."

Now, I'm flicking through a catalogue revealing a very decent selection of recent films.

"Yes, I'll have *The Last King of Scotland*, thanks."

I want to see what all the fuss was about, if Forest Whittaker really can convince as the genocidal maniac Idi Amin. More curiously, I don't quite get Scots star James McAvoy. Is he the stuff of Hollywood greats? But as one of the clinic's nurses searches for *The Last King* DVD my mind wanders and scans my own personal hair loss movie.

In the early Eighties Uncle Chris and I had talked at length about hair transplants. He revealed that Sinatra had in fact been the hair transplant pioneer, way, way, back in the early Seventies. And Frank's transplant looked great.

Or it would have done had it been real.

It transpires that Old Blue Eyes' new hair was so poor he took to wearing a wig. But he passed his wig off as a transplant, fooling the watching world into thinking he had thickening hair. But not the likes of Chris of course. And there were other sad hair stories which disappointed the world's hairless but hopeful. Television comedian Russ Abbot had a transplant in 1975 and went public with the results.

'I did it on the spur of the moment,' the TV star recalled.

'It was vanity, I suppose. I was a young drummer and wanted the hair to go with the image. Now I regret having had it done.'

Unlike Frank's head, the world did get to see Abbot uncovered – and the result was tragic. It looked as though his head had been punctured by a joiner's bridle and little tufts of hair inserted, the sort you'd see at the end of a witch's chin. If you were really being kind it looked like doll's hair.

And it was no surprise Russ chose to revert to having a bare scalp.

'The hair grew but a few years ago I decided that I wanted to go back to my natural hairline,' he said.

'And there's not a lot I can do about the scars.'

Now, as I chatted to Chris about transplants he always accentuated the positive; they will get better. They will improve. But at the time they were truly an aesthetic disaster. Early transplants involved hole punching, whereby a drill-like device would extract a plug of hair from the back of the head around 5mm in diameter, with around 20 hairs in the plug.

These were called *Standard Grafts*. Not only was this technique unsightly, the grafts, the tufts of hair were so thick that blood supply to the centre was limited and those middle hairs would die off.

If there were enough original hair around, it made the new hair bundles less visible. But of course, any surviving hair would eventually leave. And that would leave just the bundles– with the holes in the centre which the atrophied hair had occupied – standing conspicuously alone.

What also worsened the look was that the plugs were planted in stages; after the first crop, the head was left to heal for months, and then the second crop planted close to the first. But patients had to wait for the longest time before they had a head they could reveal.

A couple of years after Abbot's transplant however, there was rather more exciting new hair news. Pop idol Elton had had a procedure in Paris – and paid something like 20 grand for it. And at first I was filled with happiness. For Elton and for me. Pre-transplant, Reg would flash his pink or blond-coloured hair on *Top of the Pops* or *The Old Grey Whistle Test*. But it all looked so thin and likely to last less time than an LP. Now, with his new transplant he could look like a proper young pop star, not someone's dad.

However, post-transplant Elton took to wearing a hat. Or rather a thousand different hats. Why? Clearly he had something to hide.

'Let's see the hair, Elton!' demanded teenagers like me who had a hair worry of their own.

'We need to see the result. We need to know if it worked.'

It transpires Elton had his transplant in Paris, carried

out by France's top trichological surgeon, Dr Pierre Pouteaux. But he wasn't given plugs. According to Elton biographer Philip Norman, the pop star's new hair was down to a new and allegedly superior method of transplant called 'square grafting'.

Sections of hair bearing scalp were taken from the back of the neck, then cut into squares, and laid over the barren crown.

The advantage was that if the grafts took, growth would be faster and the covering denser than from plugs transplanted at random. The disadvantage was that several further uncomfortable operations were necessary until all the white cranial squares were filled in.

But meantime, Elton's head looked like a chessboard. Some hair was revealed a year later in a video for his new single *Ego* but the box-set transplant wasn't a success at all, no doubt hindered by the fact the pop star didn't have great donor area to begin with. So Elton covered his head with hats for years.

"Would you like some juice or anything," says Dr Farjo, as I'm thinking of Elton's head. And thinking about what Elton would have given to be able to wait thirty years before having a transplant. And not just in terms of the result. Those early transplants, as well as being unsightly, were also painful.

'When I had my hair transplants done (in 1983 and 1993) doctors said it would be mildly uncomfortable,' said techno rock icon Gary Numan much later in *The Independent*.

'Well it was horrific. They use a drill to extract thick tubes of skin and put up to 30 hairs in each hole. There's blood and it's agony. The hair all falls out to start with, which is a bit alarming, but then it grows back. About 18 months later you go back and they fill in the gaps.'

However, by 1993 the robotic-looking performer felt the procedure had improved to justify another attempt. And he allowed the clinic to use him as an advert.

'It meant I got the next treatment for free," he said. "I had the new microsurgery, (more of which later) which is much more effective and less painful.'

Numan didn't regret having had his early transplants – he regretted far more the day he told a journalist that he voted for Margaret Thatcher – but for a thinning twentysomething like me to watch these showbiz celebs emerge with these disappointing results was deflating.

Yes, it was great transplants now existed, but they were poor, The question was; when would they look good enough so's to be undetectable?

Unfortunately, those early attempts at transplanting were not the worst horror stories. Some transplants used a form of re-turfing. Doctors (if they were indeed qualified) took a long strip of hair from the back of the head but it wasn't dissected into FUs in the way it is now.

Instead, a sort of trench was dug in the scalp and the entire length of hair laid down, like a thin piece of rug being laid on a large living-room floor.

Now this was fine if you wanted to look like Chingachgook or any of the other famous Mohicans, but for most people it wasn't really ideal.

Uncle Chris even told me that some transplant surgeons would cut a flap of tissue from the side of the head on three sides, twist it and then sew it on the top.

Yes, as you can imagine, there would be a big lumpy bit. But rather than make the patient look and feel better it sounded an ideal way to torture someone.

Then there were the silicon implants. In the head. Little balloons were inserted in the skull and then gradually inflated so's to stretch the scalp. And once it had been stretched, the bald part would be cut away.

Again, a procedure you're more likely to carry out on someone you dislike a lot.

However, my hairdresser uncle kept telling me I had time on my side. That transplants would save the day.

And all I could do was hope seriously they would.

'Sure it's real. It's not mine. But it's real.'

~ **John Wayne**, when taken to task by film students, determined to connect his right-wing zeal with blatant insincerity. By way of testing him one student called out 'Is your hair real?'

4
The McQueen Crew Cut

'YES you are a very, very good doctor,' says the voice in my head.

No, it's not me projecting my thoughts on Dr Farjo's competence. The words are coming from the plasma screen. Forest Whittaker's Idi Amin is now talking to his new best friend, the young Scots doctor who has saved his life. Or rather sorted out his problem with trapped wind.

There's a strange buddy relationship going on here but I'm not really buying into it. Is it the Valium? Is it because most of my thought processes are too pre-occupied with thoughts of new hair?

Just then, the real doctor in the room interjects to tell me what he is actually doing.

"I'm removing the donor section which we'll soon be cutting into lots of follicular units," says Dr Farjo, as Amin's soldiers are also cutting open heads.

"Once we have separated them we will then implant them."

What he means by 'lots' is around 2,500 FUs. And that means around 6,000 lovely little hairs will appear on the top of my head, all made up of mostly water and keratin, constructed of 50 different proteins assembled into several layers. Fantastic. Hair will still fall out however as per the daily average. But the newly transplanted follicles will fall into the normal hair cycle of re-growth. Meanwhile, as the strip that once ran across the back of my head is being sliced, my scalp is being worked on, a series of little slits are being made on my head. My head is then washed.

"We're getting ready to implant the follicles," says Dr F, which causes me to break away from Amin and co.

"And now we are opening the scalp to allow for placement of the hair units."

What's happening is that the top of my head is being punctured with tiny blades measuring 0.7 - 0.9mm, making a series of 2,500 holes, or micro slits if you want to be scientific, into which the healthy hair follicles will be pushed.

Now, they don't have to be glued in or anything. The gap creates a sort of vacuum which sucks the FUs in. Although from what I've been reading up on post-transplant op

information, it would not be wise to go dangling upside down on a trapeze for a few weeks until they start to become attached to their new home.

Meantime, Dr Farjo has been joined by his wife, Nilofer, who is also a doctor. She will be supervising all the donor grafts being cut under the microscope as well as cutting some herself. The pair reveal that they are packing these grafts densely, at a rate of up to 50 grafts or roughly 110 hairs per square centimetre per operation, which is defined as 'ultra-refined follicular unit transplantation'.

The grafts are blended in amongst the thinning or balding areas in such a way as to match all the original growth characteristics of the original hair. Dr Farjo then explains that the follicles have to be transplanted quickly or they die, starved of blood.

Even with the Valium inside me I feel slightly anxious.

"Don't waste time talking, man. Just do it. Get them planted double quick time!"

Of course I don't actually say these words. Not to a human god who can grant me the gift of hair life once again.

And he is getting on with it. From the little pressure points on the top of my head, I'd say that he's now positioning the hair follicles. Do I feel any pain while this is all going on? Not a bit of it. And believe me, I'm the sort to whinge about a broken fingernail. Pain and me are not close friends at all.

What I'm feeling instead is someone pushing what feels like the blunt end of a pencil down on my scalp. But it doesn't bother me. What does bother me is what I'm watching on screen. Idi Amin is having even more people butchered. And still James McAvoy is unaware he's become friends with a madman!

How could this medic be so smart yet so dumb. Has he been at the morphine cupboard?

The thought takes me back to the first major medication news that gave the world's hair thinning real hope. Over the years, new information about growing new hair appeared with the regularity of spots on a teenager's chin. (And many of those cuttings made it into my personal Hairfile I had started. Just in case).

But in March, 1983 the Washington D.C. Hospital Center, announced that it was looking for volunteers to test a drug called Minoxidil's hair-growing properties. Minoxidil had originally been developed as a blood pressure medication. Inexplicably, it also grew hair on many of its users, not only on their heads, but randomly over much of their bodies.

'Most Minoxidil users weren't wild about this,' wrote

Penny Ward Moser in her article *The Bald Truth About Growing Hair* in *Discover* magazine.

'But it got Upjohn scientists to wondering. What would happen if they put Minoxidil in a lotion and rubbed it on a balding scalp? What did happen was the first real breakthrough in the quackery-riddled history of baldness "cures".' And then what happened was that the hospital came under siege, which highlighted the sheer numbers of the desperate out there who wanted hair. Badly.

And so the guinea pigs tried the solution and makers Upjohn claimed it had grown *some* hair on about 75 per cent of the users.

As is so often the case, science comes up with solutions by accident. And that was the good news. The less good news was that in about a quarter of cases, the new hair was more of a 'thin fuzz'.

But Minoxidil went on to be developed and is now sold as Regaine. And now claims it is 'clinically proven to help prevent further hereditary hair loss in four out of five men.'

Yet, it didn't seem to be the answer for me. It was relatively expensive, produced mixed results for different people - and not the amount of hair I'd hoped for.

The Minoxidil story wasn't isolated. Running parallel were the claims that scientists were coming to understand the genetics of hair and would be able to reverse the hair loss process.

But the end of the newspaper stories were always the same: the 'cures' were ten years away.

'Wish there were a cure for some of the dead cliched lines I'm having to endure watching this film,' I thought to myself as Dr Farjo continues to bring new life to the top of my head.

Just then I'm distracted by McAvoy's head. At least the Scot has good hair. Yet, I wonder how his career would have progressed if he didn't have a Hugh Grant flop?

My mind runs with the notion. There aren't too many in-your-face-baldy thesps out there. There was Yul Brynner of course. But the Swiss-Mongolian wasn't even a great actor. (Among the least convincing of *The Magnificent Seven.*) The star of that movie was of course Steve Mc-Queen - who had great hair. And all young boys in the Sixties wanted to have a Steve McQueen hairstyle.

Gosh, I've just remembered when my first Fear of Baldness moment kicked in. Something that I'd never even thought to include in the Hairfile. Just after the classic POW movie *The Great Escape* came out, I was about seven years old, I set off to have a McQueen crew cut along with my pal, Tommy McCafferty.

And so I sat there on the barber's chair (or rather on the plank of wood he used to give small boys added height) excitedly, waiting to be transformed into the insouciant, baseball-bouncing Corporal Hilts. But barber Malky Kerr had other ideas.

"Sorry, you're hair's too thin for a crew cut, son."

"Eh?"

"No can do, son."

The look on my face betrayed my utter disappointment. I wanted to look like Steve. I wanted to look American.

"I'll give you a normal hair cut," said Malky, placatingly.

And he did give me the normal short back and sides. But, and here's where the real ignominy came into play. Tommy McCafferty was then lifted onto the chair, the electric razor was pulled out and a fine crew cut administered. All for 2s 6d.

And then, to add insult to injury, Malky turned to Tommy and said, in a confident-sounding voice; "You'll never have to worry about going bald, son. Not with a head of hair like that."

"What? By implication does mean that I *do* have to worry about going bald? Eh, Malky?"

Now, to be honest, I didn't want to have hair like Tommy's. It was Post Office van red, for one thing. And it was bristly, like a new lavatory brush. Tommy was the stereotypical ghost-faced Celt.

But at least he could have a Steve McQueen.

At least he would never go bald like Yul Brynner.

And me?

'I love bald men.
Just because you've lost your fuzz
don't mean you ain't a peach.'
~ Dolly Parton.

5
Bruce's Angry Vest

RIGHT now it's 11.30am and Drs Farjo are working away pushing follicular units into my head with Korean car factory worker efficiency.

And it's a pleasing, comforting feeling. It makes me realise that while I'll never be able to have a crew cut, I won't be a Brynner.

And that gets me to thinking about contemporary actors who don't have great hair such as Billy Zane, Ben Kingsley and Jason Statham. These blokes are all prepared to go topless. They don't wear John Wayne wigs in the movies. But they play mostly psychos or hard men. And they don't get the romantic leads like Steve. None of them have ever, as far as I'm aware, got to snog Ali McGraw and Faye Dunaway.

Yes, I know some of you out there will suggest that Billy Zane managed to pull model Kelly Brooke. But that doesn't count. This is a lady who famously had to have help with reading the autocue when she was on Channel 4's *The Big Breakfast*, with tricky words spelled out for her phonetically such as 'intrepid' and 'satirical'.

Oh, I know what you're thinking; 'Who cares if she can't master three syllables - she looks great in a bikini.' Well, perhaps Billy Zane did. Deep down. As for Kingsley, without a hair piece he looks like he's about to stick a poisoned umbrella tip into someone's eye. (Except of course when he starred in *Gandhi*, but then he did have props in the form of a pair of rimless glasses, a virtual bed sheet and beatific smile to help alter his image.)

"Ouch!" I felt that last FU go in. It wasn't like being stuck with a poisoned umbrella tip but I felt it enough to take my mind off Ben. Yes, Ben. And Bruce, of course. There will be some who will argue that bald Bruce Willis looks great.

From time to time he wears a wig on film, but yes, he looks fine without hair, thanks to a strong-shaped head which looks ruggedly ok on top of a dirty vest. (Bruce's on-screen persona seems to have become angrier in direct proportion to his increasing hair loss. When did he last romance a woman on screen?)

However, while the lack of hair may give actors a decidedly angry countenance, it presents most with a serious problem. They can't run their fingers through it. Like James McAvoy is doing right now - incessantly. It's an actor's cast iron prop for conveying angst.

Brad Pitt has practically made a career out of running fingers through hair, as has Al Pacino, Andy Garcia and all of the Baldwin brothers. And how could Hugh Grant convey huge emotional distress to an audience without pushing his crowning glory backwards?

McAvoy certainly needs his hair now that Amin's Uganda is collapsing and it looks like it's time to get out of Dodge. But I'm less than concerned about the Ugandan discussions going on in front of me because I'm wandering back to the movie of my own hair loss. By my mid-thirties, I certainly didn't look Kojak-bald. Far from it. The hair hadn't packed its bags and left. It had moved on slowly, like a recalcitrant girlfriend whose heart leaves in instalments.

Like Julie, now that I come to think of it.

I was probably losing a fair bit more than the normal 25-100 hairs a day, but not enough to cause major panic. Just minor panic. And I kept a keen eye open on transplant developments.

Then one day around fifteen years ago I got the chance to see how much HT progress had been made. A Scottish TV confessional show called *Scottish Men*, a sort of *Geraldo* with Glasgow accents, announced that the theme of that week's show was Male Vanity. And the researchers of the programme had managed to uncover a young man with a new covering of hair, a hairdresser from Hamilton called Stephen.

When I heard of this intrepid young 25 year-old hair adventurer I had to interview him. However, I discovered that Stephen the Barber however wasn't just bold when it came to being effectively a guinea pig for what was very much still experimental surgery.

"How much did the transplant cost, Stephen," I queried.

"Around nine grand," he said, with a sigh.

"Well, if you don't me saying, that's a lot of money for someone to come up with." (The subtext being that 15 years ago he probably didn't earn a lot more than that in a year.)

"Yeh, you're right. The wife and I had saved up for ages to get a new fitted kitchen. And I took the money and spent it on the hair transplant."

"What?"

"Yes, I was really bothered by how I looked. And I didn't want to be completely bald so young.

"And it doesn't really do to be a bald hairdresser. (This I already knew.) For one thing you're reminded of your own situation every day. So, I spent the new kitchen money and went to London and had a hair transplant."

"And didn't your wife divorce you?"

"She threatened to," he said, laughing.

"But at the end of the day she came round. She appreciated what having hair meant to me.

"And I'm so much happier with it."

However, on meeting The Barber of Hamilton I was a little disappointed with his hair line. The result was okay. Not great. Just okay. He showed me the *Before* pics, and he was indeed close to being bald. Now, he had hair. Not thick hair, not even thick-ish hair. But a light covering that was certainly enough to take away the bare look.

And he'd had blond highlights put in. He looked like a bloke with thin, coloured hair, and it was acceptable. And it gave me some encouragement for the future.

Thankfully.

By the age of forty I wasn't tearing my hair out with worry, but I had cause for concern. It came with the realisation I was having to wash my hair every day; it needed that morning rinse to make it look more buoyant. The phrase androgenic alopecia - male pattern baldness - was now all too familiar. That's when I decided to get in touch with Malcolm. Uncle Chris had heard that techniques, particularly in Toronto, were moving forwards. Of course the www wasn't yet a search device so I contacted one of the London-based hair restoration companies that advertise regularly on the bottom right of the back page of newspapers (traditionally the most testosterone-heavy area of the paper.) And before you could say Hair Regrown In Record Time I received a letter, and an information pack, from the Senior Counsellor for the Wimpole Street Medical Practice, Malcolm Mendelsohn. Malcolm's personable letter and pack contained his own hair resume; he had had a plug transplant in 1979 - of Russ Abbott-type *Standard Grafts* - which he said looked poor after he lost his accompanying original hair.

Then he tried the hair-restoring drugs Minoxidil and Finasteride, (more of later) which gave him 'mixed results'. But in 1993 he opted for another hair transplant, this time involving *Micro Grafts*.

In the late Eighties *Mini Grafts* stopped taking the donor hair in plugs and started taking a strip, which was then sub-divided into single hairs for the hairline and mini-grafts for the other area, of 4-5 hairs.

However, the *Micro Grafts* of the early Nineties were between 1-1.5mm in diameter and had developed to the point where an even finer effect could be achieved. And this is what Malcolm had had. And it sounded really encouraging. The Sinatra-dolly head look and the Elton square days were gone for ever.

Certainly, Malcolm's results, published in the *Hair Transplant Forum International*, a monthly 'in-house publication' looked good.

Or as good as photo-copied pics can look.

But I didn't follow up Malcolm's offer to call him 'day or night' on his emergency mobile to talk about hair loss. Why? I wasn't at the point I *had* to have a transplant. And even though the hair transplant ads such as Malcolm's suggested it was a good idea to have a transplant before it was too late – so's no one would notice the contrast – that wasn't a factor for me. What was more important, I felt, was to wait until the last possible moment and allow technology to develop.

There was another factor however in not giving over my head to Malcolm. The 10 page bumph he sent out entitled *History of A Hair 'Nut'* was full of cliches and an extreme overuse of inverted commas. Worst still he committed a heinous writing crime when he described his own article *Sex, Drugs & Rock n'Roll* (explaining why he had a transplant, about how a lack of hair affected his confidence with the opposite sex) as being 'funny'. Now, I'm naturally predisposed to thinking an article is not at all funny as soon as a writer tells me it is. And it wasn't. I've since re-read Malcolm's article and I still don't understand what the Hair 'Nut' was actually talking about.

I was right to wait, as it happens. If *Micro Grafts* were the Nineties' hair transplant equivalent of the Rover-built MG sports car - decent looking for the time, but needing refinement – the current *Microscopic Follicular Units* are the Mazda MX5 – slick, stylish and reliable. For example, *Micro Grafting* didn't involve keeping FUs intact. And Micros were performed over two – or more - separate procedures. That's not the case now of course. It can all be done successfully in one sitting. I hope.

There was another difference back then compared to contemporary techniques. For a week or so the scalp would show the visible signs of the slicing and dicing it had undergone. These days, I'm assured, the slicing effects are scarcely
noticeable.

And with that thought I'm looking up at Dr Farjo and I catch his eye.

"How are you feeling there," he says.

"I'm feeling just fine."

"We're getting there," he says, reassuringly. "It's all going fine."

And just to make me feel even more fine another juice carton is placed in front of me. And a Granola Bar to nibble on.

Yes, there are worst ways to pass a day away.

"We'll be stopping for lunch in a little while."

More follicles are being pushed into my scalp. And with each push I'm feeling a little more smug.

'Thank goodness,' I thought to myself.

'No more searching for hair answers.'

The thought halts. Lunch has arrived, just in time to coincide with the end of *Last King*.

A final thought on the film slips into my incredibly busy head; 'Straight to vid.'

'How you lose or keep
your hair depends on how
wisely you choose your
parents.'

~ Edward R. Nida

6
Batboy

"HOW long will the transplant take to complete?" I'm asking Dr Farjo in between bites of a chicken sandwich.

"We should be finished around six, six-thirty," he says.

Not that time matters to me. I'm relaxed and in no hurry to go anywhere, but I have to text the Blonde with an estimated completion time. She reckons I shouldn't be alone after such a major procedure and as such has come along to lend support, to take me back to the hotel, in case I still feel a bit giddy from the effects of the Valium. At first I thought it all a bit unnecessary. But then I thought 'Why not?' She gets to play Florence Nightingale and what man can resist the chance to wallow in a bit of sympathy?

The lunch break however is also giving me the chance to think about my head. It feels numb.

"It will feel like that for a while," says Dr Farjo.

"The nerve ends will be bruised and so you won't feel much when you touch your head in some places, but the feeling will come back."

I won't be touching my head anyway, I'm thinking. Not with all those new hair follicles on it. I'll be too scared I upset one or two and they don't grow. Thankfully, I laugh at the sheer absurdity of this thought; I *know* the follicles are deeply embedded in the scalp. But all the same I don't completely suspend my own stupidity. I won't take the chance.

"Finished?" says Dr Farjo, referring to lunch. And I am. And now I'm settling down again in the big chair, this time to listen to Steve Wright on Radio 2 and the news, and I'm paying vague attention to the sports headlines. There's a story featuring former rugby player Austin Healey. A few years back he featured in lots of magazine articles after he revealed he'd recovered hair thanks to 'Advanced Hair Loss Therapy' which involved laser treatment, herbal shampoo and Minoxidil. His *Before* and *After* pics looked convincing but I wasn't convinced. I began to read up on laser therapy and couldn't build up enough evidence to suggest it would produce a great result. Nor were the *Advertising Standards Authority* completely satisfied that his hair result was down to anything but the Minoxidil. And Minoxidil, for me wasn't the answer.

Yet, transplants weren't the answer back then either. Or were they? In 2000, thanks to Glasgow Ranger manager Dick Advocaat, I began to have a re-think. The little Dutchman flew into Glasgow to continue his career with Rangers and became a hair talking point. It transpired he had had a transplant, and had spoken about it in the Dutch newspapers. The British press such as the *The Herald* and *The Independent* saw Advocaat's hair tale as a strong human interest story because here, for the first time, was a former football player owning up to having a cosmetic procedure. And admitting to feeling vulnerable.

'I've always been comfortable in my job,' he said, 'but when I had to go before the press I had to watch my hair.'

Advocaat's new hair story became the subject of a great many jokes in Scotland but he believed it was all worth it.

'I no longer need to do that,' he added of his worrying interview sessions, 'unless it is windy.'

He was also quoted as saying he'd been fed-up of being called 'kaal' – Dutch for 'bald' back at home - and decided a hair transplant would tackle that problem.

And you know what, the result wasn't fantastic – he still had a Friar Tuck bald patch - perhaps because little Dick had a football pitch-sized head to begin with, and not a lot of donor area. But it wasn't bad at all. And it offered a thought to kick around in my head.

However, what was really encouraging about the Advocaat hair experience was the fact that the football boss was prepared to open up and talk about how his baldness affected him. And thousands of bald men could empathise.

Ordinary blokes wouldn't have read the report in the *British Journal of Psychology* entitled Does Fortune Favour the Bald? It stated 'Far from being a laughing matter, male hair loss is clearly associated with a marked decrease in psychological well-being.'

It claimed bald men feel more depressed, are more unsociable and feel much less attractive. And the younger the man, the report said, the worse he felt. But they would have read the Dutchman's story. I did. And I felt part of a shared experience. Yet, I wasn't about to share his transplant experience. Not yet. For me, it was a good shot at goal but it didn't hit the back of the net.

And I had Chris telling me to hang on in there.

Meanwhile, what I did was add to the Hairfile all the stories about the wacky hair treatments that kept appearing on the market. Even though as a journalist I was born with a cynical spoon in my mouth, I was still drawn to the daft products. As a kid I was lured in by the ads I read on Page 2 of the *Superman* comics – remember the 'Genuine' X-ray specs or 'live' sea horses you could grow at home in a jar? Now, as a big boy, I found myself pulled in by magazine ads selling the electric skull caps that would stimulate the scalp by increasing blood flow, the special hair brushes, the special lamps you could shine on your head, the special electric hair brush.

I didn't buy any of course. But I have to confess I did resort to a couple of hair-saving strategies. I tried a hot oil treatment on my scalp – hairdressers had been telling me for years that I had a dry, flaky, scalp - but this didn't work either. (In fact the hot oil probably clogged my sebaceous glands' follicles up and worsened my condition.)

And I hung upside down quite a lot. Like a bat.

Why? Well, I bought a book *The Baldness Cure*, in which the basic tenet was that the head needed increased blood to grow hair. Author Andy Bryant maintained there was 'a design fault' in modern man.

'Today we are living lives which are ever more stressful, and many people run their bodies at this super-charged, battle station mode.'

Well, I could empathise with that argument.

'In doing so we affect our hair in the following ways. Because of continual stresses the blood is thicker and travels at a slower pace, finding it more difficult to enter the small capillaries once they do open again.

'Muscular tension stops the blood flow from entering and feeding the follicle.'

Sounds feasible. And he swore his 'scientifically proven' Cure really worked, which involved hanging upside down every day on a special machine, an inverter, that you could buy from him, like one of those steel traction frames you see in hospital movies. And he included photographs revealing how hair had re-grown as a result of becoming a batman. It all sounded plausible, especially when he explained the importance of diet in maintaining health hair. He even had a testimonial from MP Bryan Gould.

And I wanted to believe in the theory to the extent I barely lingered on the thought that many yoga practitioners are indeed bald.

Now, I didn't buy the special frame – I'm not *that* easily convinced – but I did take to hanging over the balcony in my hall stairs for a while. It wasn't until the Blonde came in one night and told me that the rush of blood to my head could cause me to pass out and I'd fall and break my neck and she'd be left with the organisation of my funeral, deciding who gets my guitars etc, that I realised baldness would be more preferable to death or paraplegia.

Now, here in Bessam Farjo's chair I'm wondering if my batboy adventures had continued – and I'd not fractured my spinal chord – would my hair have grown?

"Is it true that increasing the blood supply to the head encourages hair growth," I'm asking Nilofer.

"No it isn't," she says. "In fact, the opposite is the case."

"The scalp is the same all over and is usually rich in blood supply and therefore, contrary to commonly heard myths, MPB has nothing to do with lack of blood or anything else." Gosh, thank goodness I listened to the Blonde. I could have been dead – and bald.

Instead, I'm very much alive. And right now there are a rolling team of people, Bessam and Nilofer Farjo - plus the nursing team - working feverishly on my head implanting follicles to make sure that one day it will grow a fine crop of hair. This is impressive. It's like a scene from the *Elves and The Shoemaker*, with my scalp substituting for the sole of a Swiss labourer's boot.

There's a tremendous reassurance in the realisation that if there are many pairs of hands working on me constantly implanting hair, that must mean an awful lot of hair follicles are going to grow.

Two and a half thousand, in fact.

In fact it's such a comforting thought I can feel my eyes becoming heavy. I'm dropping off – in spite of the fact I'm having a procedure carried out. Is it down to the Valium? I don't think so. I think it's more down to the fact I'm contented and relaxed – and for the first time in a long time I have absolutely nothing to do but let other people take care of me. And . . .

'It's now four o'clock on Radio Two and here's some traffic news . . .'

What? Where am I. Yes, gosh, I'm in a hair transplant clinic with presenter Steve Wright and the Farjo Clinic team. Where has the time gone?

"You fell asleep for a little while," informs Dr Farjo, who for the past couple of hours has been planting.

"But don't worry, everything is going fine."

Fine. I feel fine. And it's easy to relax knowing new hair is just around the corner.

'It's a question like asking
somebody, "Did you have
breast implants?" Or "When
did you get your lobotomy?"'

~ *Star Trek* legend **William
Shatner** in response to
whether he wears a hairpiece.

7
The Tufty Club

IT'S NOW around 4.30pm and Dr Farjo and his Elves are still working away on my head, pushing FUs into my head with a passion, scarcely stopping to break.

Their effort manifests itself in a growing reassurance that I have made the right choice of surgery team, the right legion of hair superheroes to defeat the one true evil that is DHT.

So what is it? Well, since the Malcolm period I made a point of knowing exactly why a man's hair falls out. And I learned that the hair follicle has a life cycle which consists of a growing phase, a middle phase where nothing dramatic happens and a long resting phase.

A bit like a teenage boy.

It's during this resting phase, which lasts for about three months at a time (again, like the average teenage boy) that men lose hair. The hair shaft falls out and is replaced by new hair. And so the cycle continues every five-seven years.

Thankfully, each follicle acts independently - or everyone would be bald for a few months until the new hair grew in.

And that's because inside the unique hair follicle is a tiny hair factory made up of several different parts, including the hair shaft which is created, pigmented, assembled and oiled by the sebaceous glands. And it grows, appears on top of the head and then battles the elements. But the biggest battle the follicle faces is not the weather, a bad barber or even a bottle of cheap hair dye. It's a super-league bastard of a by-product called dihydrotestosterone (DHT).

If scalp hair were Superman, then DHT would be his kryptonite.

What happens is that at puberty, the testicles and adrenals secrete androgens (basically hormones) into the blood stream such as testosterone.

This testosterone enters the cells of the hair follicles, (no one knows why) where an enzyme, 5-alpha-reductase (for those science geeks who like to look things up) converts the testosterone into one of the more active androgens - called DHT.

Now, this DHT hooks itself onto a highly specific cell protein and together they stimulate the genetic transmitters that give the follicles their orders.

But that order, sadly, is the genetic equivalent of a kamikaze pilot's; the follicle is told to destroy itself. And over a period of time, (which depends upon the evil DHT instruction) the follicles begin to atrophy. The hair simply stops cycling. It hasn't the legs to continue.

Now, I know what you're thinking. If a body had no DHT there would be no hair loss. And you'd be right. It was discovered that an indigenous tribe of South American indians in Chile had no history of hair loss whatsoever. It transpires they had no DHT in their blood.

So if you were to cut off the supply of testosterone would there be no convertion to DHT? Yes, that would be the case. And it's been highlighted over the centuries that those men who have been castrated don't have a problem with hair loss.

However some may consider this a little extreme.

And it may not even offer a guarantee. Although the bulk of male androgens are produced by the testicles, they are also produced by the adrenal cortex. This is why transsexual women who were born men, even though they've had their genitals removed their adrenals supply enough testosterone to cause their hair to fall out.

"Gosh, so even if I had become a transsexual, the DHT could still have got me."

Thankfully, I didn't say that sentence loudly enough for Dr Farjo to hear me.

Instead, I rewind once more on my hair loss history, to the point where it had all became rather dramatic. By the age of 45 I was buying hair-thickening shampoos. And they worked, to a degree.

What they helped me to do, these shampoos called *Big Volume* or *Bubblehead* or whatever, was to look in the mirror and somehow convince myself I didn't have a major problem with baldness. And thanks to the fact that I had enough hair on the front there was at least the illusion of quantity.

Yes, I was in denial - highlighted one day by my reaction to being invited onto a BBC radio programme to discuss hair loss. There had been a news report out that week about a new solution that could help grow hair. And so the producer came up with the idea of a debate about whether or not men should graciously accept the parting of the parting. "Why me?" I quizzed the producer. (Now, he didn't know that I had been compiling notes and bits of information on hair loss and possible cures for years, stuffed away in my cardboard Hairfile.)

"Because you can talk on the subject."

"I can blether about most subjects. But why me"

"Well, em, you are, a little, em, follicly challenged."

"Mmm. Well, perhaps a little."

And so I appeared on the show. And the position I adopted, loosely, was *Why Should Anyone Be Happy Being Bald If They Don't Have To Be? - Drink Paraffin If It Will Bring Your Hair Back.*

And it was quite an experience.

Others on the programme – including one female journalist - cited the usual old tosh about how some men embrace baldness. And how some women love some men who are bald.

And, yes, the old bald chestnut himself Sean Connery was tossed onto the fire of debate.

However, Sir Sean was quickly hauled off again after I asked the question 'If the world loves Shone's hairless head so much why has he not appeared in a single movie since *The Man Who Would Be King* without a hairpiece?'

And I went on to quote a list of movie stars who concealed the bald truth, from Fred Astaire to Ted Danson to Frank Sinatra.

One (bald) contributor argued that a man with thinning hair should simply shave it all off.

"Be a man!" he said, as his glove slapped hard against my cheek. My reply was that this indeed was a much preferable solution to the problem than relying upon the tried and lambasted Donald Trump/Bobby Charlton/Ron

Atkinson comb-over technique. But, I maintained if a real 'cure' for baldness *did* appear why not take advantage of it? With a hairline, I argued, men look ten years younger.

"Yes, but that's just vanity."

"Isn't everything we do to keep ourselves looking good about vanity? Buying an Armani suit, getting a good hair cut, having our teeth fixed?"

"That suggests men are becoming more like women," said the female reporter.

"Isn't it rather sexist to say that self-improvement should be the sole preserve of the female sex?" I countered.

The post-debate callers to the show reckoned I had won out. But it wasn't a total victory. Some men simply believed that even considering a hair treatment was too much of a trip to Vanity Central. The radio debate was academic however. The solution which had formed the peg for the piece was later discovered to be ineffective. There was no *real* solution to the problem of re-creating a full head of hair. You can't turn back nature.

But appearing on the programme made me look in the mirror a little more closely. And worry. Would a transplant work now? I searched the websites for results, and came up with a blurb featuring the world's most famous headbanger, Status Quo's Francis Rossi. He cited his reasons for getting a transplant in *The Sun*. In two words. 'Phil' and 'Collins'.

'I was aware of it (the hair loss) because I remember people getting me and Phil Collins confused and I didn't like that.' Now, this may seem rather an extreme reason for getting a transplant. Phil seems a nice enough bloke and he's not bad looking. But the Quo frontman's claimed need not to be mistaken for the Genesis singer was enough to see him undergo a procedure at the Wellesbourne Hair Transplant Clinic.

'Francis has had three procedures in total and was so pleased with his treatment that he went public, discussing his reasons for hair transplantation in newspapers, TV and radio,' says the blurb by Dr Rogers.

'His hair now looks like it did in 1986, for the Status Quo hit *Marghuerita Time.*'

Mmm. I looked at the pics of the hair-swinging rock star back in '86 and his post HT photos and his new hair didn't look as if it could be combed, never mind swung from side to side. Or perhaps I'd had a few too many marghueritas at the time.

Sure, Francis had more than he had before the procedure - a little at the front grown long and combed backwards into a pony tail - but I wasn't overly impressed. There wasn't a great deal going on up there.

It turns out Rossi had had three procedures to get this thin landing strip of hair. After being in the chair three times I'd expect to have real rock star hair planted and growing. Like Led Zeppelin's Robert Plant in fact.

But perhaps the Quo frontman didn't have a great donor area. That said, the musician was delighted with the result. Or he wouldn't have gone public. And transplant surgeon Dr Rogers was quoted in the *Sunday Mirror* as saying how pleased he was with the results of the procedure - and revealed he has in fact treated other members of the band. Dr Rogers then spoke about how much the technique had improved in recent years.

'In the past men had their head ruined with punch grafts,' he said.

'Surgeons would take 4cm pieces of scalp from the back of the head. Then put them in holes the same size at the front. This caused scaring if the grafts didn't take and often left a bizarre tufty effect.'

Well, at least the Tufty Club has now closed for good. And transplants do work. They do. Not all that fantastically for ageing three-chord rock stars, if his pics are anything to go by, but they do work.

They do, I kept telling myself, more in hope than certainty.

And I failed to be entirely convinced again when I saw actor John Cleese's transplant result of 1989.

'I redistributed my hair on socialist principles,' he joked at the time. And while the joke wasn't that funny at least he was bold enough to own up to his procedure. (More of which later.)

Again, it looked ok. But nothing more. Yes, my faith in the transplant ever being the perfect solution was starting to weaken. But what was a hair melodrama in my Thirties became a Sam Raimi horror in my late Forties. One day I queued up in a garage to pay for petrol - and got a real shock. It wasn't the cost of fuel – the price hadn't exploded at that stage – the scare came about when I caught sight of myself on CCTV.

For the first time in a very long time I saw what the top of my head looked like. And at first, I couldn't believe it was my attached to my body. I wanted it to be someone else's. But after moving my body around, I realised the image on the camera also moved. And I looked hard at the reality. I had very little hair on my crown.

It really *was* time to think about the options. In recent years I had looked closely at my diet, I had cut down on sugar which was one of the things Chris had suggested.

But there was nothing I could do it seems about the effects of DHT.

"Ouch!" a little sharp prick stops my meandering thoughts. One particular follicle insertion isn't sliding in like the rest for some reason and a little extra pressure is being applied. It hurts. Okay, I'm a cry baby. It *would* have hurt had it been five times as sore and my head not anaesthetised.

Where was I? Yes, the garage incident. Which led me to look closer at the bald truth. For years I had been reading that American companies were spending billions on cracking the hardest of all nuts, the hairless nut. It was the Holy Grail of US drug companies. Would they find it soon? I needed it soon.

I began to look more closely at the hair treatment ads strategically placed on the back pages of newspapers. They all offered the world in the form of better hair.

Footballers such as Celtic star John Hartson were lining up to lend their not inconsiderable weight to the likes of 'new laser surgery' - and claiming great results.

Unfortunately, Hartson's results on the pitch were better than the contest he was having with his departing hair follicles. When I watched the ginger striker play in an Old Firm match, for once I was not interested in his performance. I was looking closely at his scalp. His hairless scalp. Once again, laser didn't cause my face to beam.

Other ads featuring sports stars however looked more promising. Cricketers such as Graham Gooch revealed their hairline had been saved. And the photographic evidence certainly looked good. But I felt stumped after reading more about the companies involved. It seemed the results were down to hair weaving.

Yes, hair weaving. That's what Elton has today. And the thin, warbly-voiced Robin from the Bee Gees. And several big name Hollywood actors, according to the showbiz websites. Mind you, the results looked good. And Captain Fantastic's head looks, well, fantastic.

But when I read up on weaves and how fake hair is joined to existing hair with clips and knots and pulled through a mesh it didn't seem the answer for me. It was all a bit too industrial. (Yet, not an option I was prepared to discard totally.)

I needed hope. Real hope that real, growing Cassidy hair would one day appear on my head.

'I have pale blue eyes and I was receding in my late twenties.
And if you look like this and you're twenty-eight you play rapists.'

~ Actor **Patrick Malahide.**

8
Don King

TWO years ago, on my 50th birthday - what better time to make a life-changing decision? - I stepped up the effort to recover my head.

The phrase 'hair-parting' had suddenly taken on a whole new meaning for me.

And to be honest, by this time the hairline was thinner than Agyness Deyn's thong.

From the front of my head there was just enough fuzz to take away the bare look, to allow me to live in denial. But the reality was I was almost topless. I had to take action. But what sort?

I was ready to look at every option again. And then one arrived, funnily enough, at Glasgow Airport Arrivals. My close pal for the past 30 years, Aidan, who's an actor, came up to visit for a couple of days.

And as I waited for him at the airport I caught sight of him on the security screens. The first thing I noticed was that he seemed to have more hair. He had a full fringe. Not quite a Ringo Starr c1964 fringe, but certainly a neat little curtain of hair at the top of his head. And I smiled knowingly as he walked into the terminal.

"You look great," I said, grinning.

"Thanks," he said, smiling.

"Ok. What have you done to your hair?"

"I've had a weave," he said. "I found I was going up for parts of blokes in their early forties. But the thinning hair made me look older. So I did something about it. And I like it. No one can tell."

He added, laughing; "Except you. But then you did spend a lot of time with your Uncle Chris."

He was right. But his new hair did look great. A few weeks later we had a night out with the partners and I didn't mention my pal's weave to the Blonde at all. She was clueless.

And I know I had previously dismissed fake hair coverings as an option, but now I began to re-run the weave possibility over in my head.

Should I think about an Elton? – the new Elton hair answer, that is.

Later, I watched Aidan (not his real name) on stage in the West End alongside thousands of people and none would have had a single thought that his hair wasn't his own.

"It looks fantastic," I said afterwards.

"But what does it feel like on your head?"

"It feels normal. I don't think about it. Unless of course I get a bit of teasing from the wife about it."

"Can I touch it?"

"Sure."

And I did. He let me touch his scalp. And I could feel the ever-so-slight bump of the silicon ridge into which the hairs are inserted.

And I could imagine me touching this ridge every

minute of every day it was on my head.

And because I'd be aware I'd assume other people *may* be aware. Oh dear. And on top of that, the hair topping costs £60 a month for 'maintenance'. I didn't like the idea of being maintained.

No, a weave wasn't an option for me. So I looked for a solution. Literally. Now there was the likes of new improved Minoxidil-based *Regaine* on the market, but I didn't feel the difference on using it would be that dramatic.

And at this time another pal, co-incidentally also an actor (note; my social circle includes those who are not thespians) told me he was taking Finasteride and was getting good results.

Finasteride, originally prescribed to treat prostate enlargement, works by preventing testosterone from converting into DHT.

I could see it was working. He didn't have hair in abundance. But it was thicker than it had been a year back and looked good. (I'm absolutely sure he'd be bald right now if he hadn't used it.) There is however a two per cent chance of side effects (possible impotence) with drugs such as Finasteride, although these can disappear if you persevere.

Now it so happened that a friend of his, who is also thinning, had tried Finasteride. And sadly, he'd gone a bit floppy.

No, it wasn't for me. So I searched the net and discovered a company who were offering to re-grow your own hair using stem cells. This sounded fantastic. We'd all known for years that the world's illnesses (and hairloss) would one day be cured by stem cells, nature's building blocks. Back in the early Eighties, Colin Jahoda, now of Durham University, published a paper detailing how he had induced new rat whiskers to develop and grow from cultured cells.

This early rat whisker's success could now be the cat's whiskers as far as the world's hairless were concerned. And over the years stem cell developments continued.

But there were a couple of problems with this particular stem cell 'cure.' The first was that the company was based in Mexico. Why Mexico? Is Mexico the epicentre of stem cell research? I didn't think so.

Then there was the cost. At $30,000 it sounded a little expensive for cultivating a few cells in a jam jar. But there was another price to pay.

Side effects.

Latin American scientific reports claimed the stem-celled hair would grow in one colour only – white – and in any direction it chooses.

I didn't want to look like Don King.

'Balding is God's way of showing you are only human. He
takes the hair off your head and
sticks it in your ears.'

~ **Bruce Willis**

9

The Hair Raising Search

NOR did I want to look like James Taylor. Sweet Baby James yes, but not the JT I saw perform in Glasgow.

The legend sounded wonderful but looked a little worn without his Seventies hippy-style hair. And I felt worn too. To have hair like David Cassidy again - that's the dream.

Yet, it seemed the only way to achieve that dream was to have a transplant. But only if they had come a long way.

Sadly, little Uncle Chris was no longer around to advise. At just 72 he'd played his last ever game of football.

And so I looked around at the hundreds of clinics offering to transplant my hair. And many looked entirely convincing.

And slowly but surely my search developed into a Freddie Krueger of a nightmare. I discovered thousands of websites offering information on hair treatment centres, based, it seemed in every corner of the globe but mostly in the States.

And there were hundreds of thousands of testimonies to read.

But could I take the word of a 23 year-old from Alabama who recounts his own 'true-life' experience? How did I know he hadn't gone to a shack in the woods to be treated by a doctor who's last job was removing swamp ticks?

How did I know he didn't once date his sister?

The internal debate in my head about the relative merits of transplant - not about relative relations - continued for some time.

Meanwhile, it's now 5.30pm, and the Drs Farjo are still filling my head with recycled hair, working tirelessly, and all is going well.

I'm massively impressed with the effort, considering this is a daily occurrence for them. And I have a great sense of well-being. I'm completely relaxed, so much so that my mind drifts back to my dilemma of whose hands to place my head in.

The title of a song by the great Hairgod himself, Cassidy, constantly filled my head back; *How Can I Be Sure*?

I considered 'touching base' with Malcolm again but his over-use of the inverted commas had stayed with me. However, the more I read the true-life hair experiences on the many internet sites the more I was confused. For every nine great results it seemed there was always one story that could easily have formed the basis for a Hammer Films script.

I needed A Sign, something which confirmed that transplants could guarantee a Doris Day ending. Then one day I met a pal, Jack, for coffee and to talk about a TV idea. We took to chatting about my hair dilemma and he revealed to me he'd been doing a lot of research into the subject of hair loss, just to keep his own barnet in good working order.

He told me I had to read Spencer Kobren's book, *The Bald Truth*. And that should provide some of the answers to my questions. And I did. And a terrific little book it was too. Kobren, a young American, wrote honestly and independently of his Stateside adventures in desperately seeking a baldness cure.

'I had been literally counting hairs and saving them in plastic bags and labelling them to compare weekly counts (C'mon, we've all been there, right?),' he admits.

Kobren had looked at all the options. And while he went for the Finasteride solution, and got a very good result, he concluded that transplants were highly possible - and practical. And a one-off expense.

He confirmed that the days when heads were left looking like World War 1 French battlefields were long gone. The modern hair follicle transplantation process had come of age.

The first major breakthrough had come about in 1984 when a pathologist discovered that hair grew in clusters of 1-4 units. Then in the late Eighties an American, Dr Bobby L. Limmer introduced the use of the microscope in HT surgery which meant that hair could be more easily dissected into the tiny units.

But it wasn't until 1995, writes Kobren, that hair transplant surgery 'took a huge leap forward.' The process was refined by using microsurgery with small hair units. But it wasn't just about taking small groups of hair and moving them from donor site to the top of the head. It was about taking the *right* groupings of hairs and transplanting them. Follicular transplantation had arrived.

I liked the way Kobren had presented the evidence.

And he didn't use inverted commas at all.

But if hair transplants could now produce great results, there was still a major hurdle to leap. Kobren and all the website comments said the same thing; HTs can still go horribly wrong. You *have* to have the right surgeon.

What's paramount to achieving a successful hair transplant is the skill of the surgeon, someone who can work at speed with tiny hair units comprising of one-four hairs - which have then to be inserted undamaged and lined up properly into the slits already made on the scalp.

And they have to be able to stitch up the back of the head, without it looking like it's been done by a First Year Home Economics student who's desperate to get home to Facebook pals she's only just left.

So how do you find the right man for the job? Do you have to go to the United States or Canada? It's not that I wasn't prepared to go to such lengths to have long hair again, but was it necessary?

Most of the on-line testimonies were by Americans. And while I like many of them I confess to a general mistrust of citizens of a country only 10 per cent of whom hold a passport, have never seen an ocean, deify *Geraldo* and have voted two Bush men into office.

I called one of the UK's top trichologists for independent advice. He, or rather one of his assistants, relayed the info that you don't in fact have to go to the States to get a great hair transplants, which was reassuring. But he then recommended his 'own transplant surgeon' - which didn't sound that independent to me.

And so I made a few more calls to cosmetic clinics around the country. And I spoke to lots of sales people who all promised they could make me hairier than a Greek grandmother's top lip – without having seen sight of my head.

Mmm. I needed to do more research.

I read up on the hospitals in Buenos Aires which were offering cheap transplant deals. And they were cheap - around a third of the price you were expected to pay in the UK. And the idea of returning to a city I'd once adored had great appeal.

But if something sounds too good to be true . . .

Then I spoke to the Harley Street company offering a new transplant technique whereby rather than dissecting a strip taken from the back of the head, a device is used to pulls the follicles out and re-plant them in the front. *Follicular Unit Extraction* was its Sunday name.

It sounded great. And I liked the idea of not having a strip of scalp removed. So I went down to London to this clinic to check it out.

What I got to see was the waiting room I was ushered into. And as I waited I sat alone, apart from an unsmiling man of around sixty who wore a suit that didn't seem to sit comfortably upon him.

After about five minutes I was then led into a small white-walled office by a female of indeterminate accent and vague job description. She opened a laptop and showed me CGI images of a bald head. Then she showed the same head again, but this time with hair. Mmm.

Was she a doctor? No, a 'company manager'. I assumed she was essentially a saleswoman. The lady then produced a video programme that counts hairs on heads, scanned over my own head with what looked like a brush with a light on and now my head was on her computer. She then estimated how many follicular units I would need.

"You would need around 3,000," she said. "But I think you would be a very suitable candidate for treatment be-cause you have a very good donor area."

Great. And she told me the cost. It was expensive, around £3 a unit. But I could go to Greece she said and get it done 'much cheaper'. Well, it sounded interesting. But I didn't commit myself.

"What's the name of the doctor who would perform the transplant?" I asked. "It depends," she says. "We use a pool of doctors."

"Can't you be specific?"

"No, not at this time. Not really."

Aside from creating an image in my head of a group of surgeons splashing around wearing water wings, I decided her answer didn't work for me. I needed to know the name of a surgeon so I could check his credentials.

Spencer Kobren would have been shocked to learn I'd done otherwise.

Now I have to say I didn't get a hard sell from the lady - more a contrived indifference. I felt she was saying to me 'Well, we know you'll be back because you have no choice'.

But I wasn't sure about her company at all. I wasn't convinced. However, just as she finished giving me the cost details, the sales lady had another card to play.

She asked me to wait a moment as she ushered in 'someone you should meet.'

It was the bloke with the suit from the waiting room. He'd had a hair transplant, she said. And this suit bloke had indeed. And it looked fine. The hairline looked fairly natural. But I wasn't sure at all I should sign on the line which was dotted. I felt the process was all too mechanical, too cold. And I really needed to know the name of the doctor who'd work on my head.

So I tried other clinics in the UK who claimed terrific

hair transplant results. And one, with centres in the North West, the Midlands and London sent out a brochure so expensive-looking I reckoned it would take the cost of ten hair transplants to produce it.

Yet, there were points in this work of art that caught my attention. It pointed out that hair transplantation was '80 per cent artistry and 20 per cent surgical skill'.

Mmm. I guess it is hugely important that the surgeon had an eye for the aesthetic, the ability to get the hairline just right.

And it listed the prices, in the same range as the Harley Street clinic. What I didn't take to however were the photos of oak-paneled desks set in thick-carpeted office suites. I reckoned the place was making far too much money. And I wasn't too keen on the first *Before* and *After* pics to confront me. They were of a man in his late thirties and if someone told me he was a Cuban drug dealer with a couple of felony raps I'd have believed them.

Gosh, this guy looked serious, and shifty, thanks to a starey-eyed expression, a slicked back hairstyle and a sharp goatee beard. But it was the pony tail that really put me off.

Look, I know what you're thinking, it's the hair density that I should have been focusing upon. And you're right. But a hair transplant is about more than that. It's about looking right. It's about buying into a wonderful hair dream. And this bloke looked a little too intimidating.

Now, if he'd been a David Cassidy look-alike . . .

As a result of reading the big, full-colour brochure I was left frustrated.

What to do? I wondered what Malcolm is up to? Okay, I know the whole inverted commas thing put me off, but he did sound incredibly committed to the hair-saving process. I wondered if he had something new to offer?

A look on his website revealed that Malcolm was now part of a company that used the 'Choi' Implanter Technique. And it was hard to work out how it worked, but it seemed a large needle was used to extract the follicles from the donor area and then implant them onto the front of the head.

To be honest, I didn't read on in any great depth because the 'Choi' technique involved going to Athens ('it's far too labour intensive for the UK') and the surgeon and his 'large team of assistants' were unnamed.

I had to smile though when I read the website blurb. It had Malcolm's 'mark' all over it.

'Being 'needle' work, 'Choi' work is a lot safer. The healing 'spot' is literally that, a small blood spot which wastes away within four or five days. In fact the surgery site is so 'neat' as to not draw attention.'

Enough of the inverted commas, Malcolm.

So I was back where I started. One day however hope appeared in the form of our office secretary, Janice. We'd got talking about my disappearing hair and she told me that her friend's husband's brother had had a hair transplant. And the result looked 'pretty good'.

"Great, Janice. Ask him if he'll give me a ring."

Two weeks later, nothing.

"Well, can I give him a ring?"

"He doesn't want to talk to you."

"Why?"

"Cos' you're a journalist, I guess."

"I'm not going to write about him. I don't even need to know his real name. He can call himself Zorro if he likes.

I just want him to tell me what went on on his head. And where. And who did it. And how much."

"I'll ask again."

And nothing. Clearly, this bloke wanted to keep the secret of eternal hair life to himself.

'The rotten selfish bastard,' I thought in a moment where magnanimity was harder to find than a solid recommendation.

So close - and yet so far from the hair apparent.

Then suddenly the answer was staring me in the face.

'It is foolish to tear one's hair
in grief, as though sorrow would
be made less with baldness.'

~ Marcus T. Cicero.

10
Man From Uncle Hair

"YOU should go and see Dr Farjo," said TV Dragon and multi-millionaire businessman Duncan Bannatyne.

No, the Scot with the £300m fortune and irascible persona didn't offer this advice to me directly. It came to me when the star of TV's *Dragon's Den* appeared on popular ITV show *Fortune: Million Pound Giveaway,* where ordinary people ask the millionaires panel for money for a variety of reasons, usually altruistic.

However, in a February 2007 episode one bold, thick-skinned and thin-haired young man stepped forward and asked for money for a hair transplant. For himself.

Duncan Bannatyne then asked this young man if he had consulted with Dr Farjo! He added; 'Dr Farjo is the best, no one will ever know you had it done!'

As you would expect, the media picked up on this. Including me. Had Duncan Bannatyne had a hair transplant? Was he making this recommendation based on personal experience? Seems he was. Regardless, I had to find out who this Dr Farjo was, this man who came with such a high profile champion. And thanks to Google, the answer was revealed in seconds. Dr Farjo turned out to be one of the most eminent transplant surgeons in the UK. Both Dr Bessam and his wife Nilofer Farjo are Fellows of the Institute of Trichologists, Fellows of the European Academy of Cosmetic Surgery and Founder members of The Trichological Society etc, etc.

Dr Farjo, I discovered, had carried out over 4,000 hair transplants. So it wasn't hard to see why the Scots businessman chose to have a hair transplant at the Farjo Clinic.

Right about this time however, a newspaper carried an interview with Sean Williamson of *Extras* fame. So what? Well, when he was Barry in BBC soap *Eastenders* the actor was as bald as Bilko. Now, he has hair. It's not thick, floppy Hugh Grant hair, but he's not bald. And it looks great, especially when you consider that he had an area the size of Walford to cover. And it transpired he'd had his transplant at the Farjo Clinic.

Was the Farjo Clinic the answer to my own marble head? I called the next day and spoke to the manager, Mick. He was pleasant and seemed genuine. How can you tell? After 30 years of asking questions for a living you just know. And there's that feeling you get when you like someone straight off.

So I decided to go down and look at the Farjo set up, a state-of-the-art but not overly flash-looking clinic right in the heart of Manchester's Picadilly.

I discovered Mick to be as likable in the flesh. But just as importantly, he spoke for as long as it took to explain the process, about how long it would take, how I would feel the next day, what sort of result I could expect.

His replies were understated – he never used hyperbole, but nor was he distant, like he were selling me a bathroom suite. I got the feeling he loved the work he did and loved the idea of balding men having new hair.

Then he introduced me to Dr Bessam Farjo, a man with a genial persona and a relaxed manner. Dr Farjo asked me what I'd be hoping for in terms of new hair, no doubt wondering would my expectation far out weigh the reality. Did I hope to end up with Orlando Bloom locks? When I pointed out that I didn't (I never even hinted at my Cassidy dreams) there was a detectable smile of relief on his face. I sensed that some prospective clients assume they will look like they did as a teenager again. But without the platform shoes and the acne.

Dr Farjo then produced a black felt pen, and he asked if he could draw on my head.

"What, a Popeye cartoon?" I asked, grinning.

And so he did. Not the Popeye cartoon but an outline of where my new hair outline would grow, should I agree to go ahead with the process.

And you know, it looked pretty much as I'd hoped it would – not too square across the top, which I knew would look unrealistic, but offering enough to take away the bald look.

To be honest, I don't think there's anything wrong with the temples showing, just so long as there's that archipelago of hair at the front to catch the eye; I'm thinking Robert Vaughn in his *Man From Uncle* days.

But as well as being realistic, Dr Farjo's drawing, or rather the black ink he'd drawn on my head, had the effect of giving me the illusion of hair. It was a little insight of what it could be like one day.

And the future, with hair, was a seductive prospect.

Then I got to ask all the relevant questions; how long

does the procedure take? (An entire day). Do you have instant hair? (No, it will start to grow in after three to four months). Will there be much scarring when the follicles are implanted? (None). How thick will it be? (A good covering). Can it fall out? (No.) How many hairs will I need. (Around 2,500 follicular units). Will I become more attractive to the opposite sex and have 28 year-olds chasing me round the disco? (Unlikely. And be careful of what you wish for.)

Then I told him about a concern, about a businessman I spotted on a plane, not so long ago and it was obvious this bloke had had a transplant. Why? Well, he didn't have too much hair on top – he had rather a big area to cover, but the new hairline was perfectly formed. And it looked like a perfect row of little hairs all on a perfect line. It was like going to a garden centre to buy a Christmas tree to discover a front row of perfect little trees all lined up, but only scraggly ones spaced out behind them.

This didn't encourage me at all have my own new little forest.

"That result is down to the way the hairs were implanted," said Dr Farjo.

And so he explained his planting process, of one, two, three and four hairs units, because that's they way they grow naturally in your head.

"By mixing up the amounts and placing them correctly we get as close to reality as possible."

In order to create this naturally haphazard effect on my head, Dr Farjo said he would map out the area like a grid reference and hair shafts allocated appropriately.

Now, the scalp has around 100,000 hair follicles, or some 1,000 per square inch. (Blondes can have up to

140,000, but they tend to produce thinner hair. Brunettes have 110,000 follicles, redheads 90,000.)

And I was never going to get to anything like the 1,000 per square inch figure (not that I had that density to begin with).

However, there was real hope of real cover. Aha. The trick is to plant the hair in a way that it doesn't look as if it's been grown in a greenhouse.

"That's the plan," said Dr Farjo, smiling.

I liked him. More importantly, I trusted him. He didn't have a great head of hair himself - which raised a question in my head. (I learned later he'd had a transplant, but didn't have sufficient donor area thickness, which is rather ironic, considering his ability to re-cover others.)

But he gave me all the time I needed to explore all the issues. And he offered to put me in touch with men who had had a transplant and lived locally.

I felt confident in his ability but, just as importantly, I felt he had a personal interest in me.

"You won't get a thick head of hair," he said, "but you have good growth area at the back and we can transplant it to the top and get a decent result."

I was convinced. But back with Mick for a final chat he insisted I go away and think about it. And I did, for at least a couple of weeks. And I called Mick back. And I spoke to him about the London clinic and FUE method, know in the business as 'plug and tug'.

"We also use the FUE method," said Mick.

"But on very selective cases.

"However, we don't feel it works so well where a great deal of follicular units need to be transferred and where we are aiming to do a one-off procedure. You see, this sys-

74

tem involves the individual follicular units being manually extracted using on average 1mm 'drill bits'.

"So instead of one fine-line scar, there will be a large number of very small dot scars and these are spread along the whole donor area. One issue for patients is that often the donor region has to be shaved down to allow easier access for the surgeon. It's a lot more time consuming and therefore more limited in the number of grafts possible to transplant in a session. Therefore it's going to be more expensive.

"The other problem with it is in the extraction of hairs. Sometimes hair follicles grow at an angle. And with the 'plug and tug' method, you may not get the follicle intact. We reckon that there's around a 10-20 per cent loss of follicles during extraction using this method."

"I don't fancy those statistics," I said. "I want every hair removed from the back to be in first class condition to face a new life on top."

"Exactly," said Mick. "You want to maximise your donor area. In our opinion, the FUE method may be appropriate where a small number of hairs are required, such as with eyebrows, or where the strip method isn't possible due to extensive previous transplants.

"Or if someone wants an extremely short hair cut and prefers not to have a line scar. And FUE could be used to refine old-style plug surgery." And I came to a conclusion. It seemed to me that with Dr Farjo's credentials, high-profile recommendations and straight-talking - combined with his manager's likable, empathetic manner - my head was in safe hands.

"Let's go for it!" Mick.

'I don't have any sperm left. If I stop taking the pills, all my hair will fall out. But I would rather have hair than sperm.'

~ **Rupert Everett,** on the baldness medication that may reduce his tadpole count.

11
The Aged Asbo

AND now here I am. And it's six o'clock and I'm a little surprised the process is taking quite so long.

Yet, I'm relaxed, sipping another juice and chewing on a piece of Granola bar. Every now and then I become aware of an FU being pushed into my head but for the most part I just lay back and think of the recent build up to this moment. After talking to Mick and setting a date for the transplant, the concerns kicked in. There was a fear of the procedure itself of course, agreeing to have a twelve inch-long and half-an-inch wide strip of my head removed - given that most people are so terrified of the side effects of surgery.

And I'd seen the American website photographs which revealed examples of where the strip technique had gone horribly wrong, with Frankenstein-like stitches running across the back of some poor guy's head.

I'd read all about the cosmetic surgery disasters, the reports about footballer Colin Hendry's wife who almost died after she had a tummy tuck. And I'd read countless newspaper stories about how infections can be picked up so easily. But I managed to put the worries aside; I thought of Spencer Kobren's mantra which maintained that HT success was all about the right surgeon.

And I believed I'd made the right choice. And right now I'm smiling at the fact this is hardly a Victorian hospital ward I'm sitting in; more a state-of-the-art-scrubbed-'till-it-bleeds clinic that I'm convinced laughs in the face of cryptosporidium sores.

There were other concerns however. I wasn't sure about the reaction I'd get from other people. Telling friends and family what I was planning to do was a big hurdle.

I remember once reading a feature in the *Daily Mail* in which thinning writer David Thomas had considered all the hair replacement options - wigs, weaves and transplants. And he'd decided, although hating the idea of being bald, not to go for any of them.

It was an informative and very funny piece. However, he wrote one line which stuck in my head; (and remained there, having soon been transferred to the Hairfile).

'My wife swears she has no problem with my hair-loss. If I ever bought a toupee or had a hair transplant she'd throw me out of the house.'

Wow! That's a bit drastic. But it got me to thinking that perhaps some people simply abhor the idea of a bloke getting new hair.

I once tested this theory. I threw the possibility of me having a hair transplant out in the direction of a girlfriend - and she threw it right back in my face.

"That's just not what men do," she said, reprovingly.

I was taken aback. She'd reacted as though I'd told her I was in advanced stages of gender realignment, planning to buy a Laura Ashley frock, a pair of Manolo Blahnik kitten heels and a subscription to *Marie Claire*.

I guess from her point of view she was shocked, that a

man, whom she thought she knew fairly well, could be so vain and so, well, girlie. (Of course metrosexuality hadn't been invented at that time.)

Suddenly, I wasn't a bloke who could fit a new kitchen or sort out a blocked drain (not that I was to begin with, but she hadn't had the chance to discover this).

Instead, I was a self-obsessed, preening peacock.

However, in the past few months female friends were supportive. Brenda and Lesley thought it a great idea. And both suggested I write about the experience. Perhaps not surprisingly since they are both journalists.

Thankfully, the current partner, the Blonde, was happy about it. She had listened to me throw the idea around for so long she wasn't surprised when I firmed it up.

In fact, I reckon it was something of a relief for her to know it was finally going to happen; I'd stop talking about it. And part of her was with me in attempting to end for all time, hopefully, the bald jokes that would creep into conversation towards the end of parties when blokes were so drunk they felt they could be brave.

My family were fine, overall. My mother worried if it would be 'sore', and if there were a medical risk attached. And I said no more than going into hospital to have a skin blemish removed.

My daughter Nat was also positive about my hair dream. And some close pals were entirely supportive.

"You've always been a vain bastard," said old university chum Steve, now living in Australia.

"But that's easy for me to say because my hair is okay. Just grey. And I think you should get it done. It will make you feel better."

Writer pal Ian's attitude was simply I didn't need to have

it done. "I don't see you as bald," he said. "Your hair looks okay."

"Yes, but the hair I have left has a life of about six months. After that, there'll be nothing left on top."

"You'll suit it," he maintained. "You don't need to have a hair transplant."

Robert, an irascible impresario with very thick hair, was a little more resolute.

"You don't f****** need it!" he exclaimed.

"You're eight years older than me and you look five years younger. Save your money. Or give it to me!"

Davy, who's an electrician, and has little hair himself, said 'Go for it.'

Jim however, who runs a housing empire, and who has very little hair left, was pretty much against the whole idea.

"Just shave it all off like I do," he says. "Get yourself a good razor and set it to Number 2. It'll look fine."

"No Jim, because I will look like an aged Asbo or an axe murderer."

"No you won't. And some people look good bald."

"Yes, six feet-four African-American basketball players. And my ultimate tennis hero, Andre. And my old, well-built tennis pal Mark seems to wear it well. But not five foot seven and a half inch Oor Wullie-skinned Scots."

Jim was arguing the case for empowerment; don't wait for Mother Nature to take away what's left of your hair topping, do away with it yourself. And I could see where he was coming from. Make yourself believe that you are choosing to be bald.

"The only problem with that Jim, is I don't choose to be bald. I don't look good with very short hair and I will look even less good with no hair whatsoever.

"In fact, I will look like I've just emerged from one of Her Majesty's Institutions, having been in there in the first place for a very serious crime."

"You won't! Be a man. Get it shaved."

"No Jim. I may never have a David Cassidy hairline again. It may not even be Butch Cassidy. But at least it won't be Butch Wilkins."

But while blokes like Jim argued the case for revealing the bald truth, I couldn't forget my memories of Chuck. Chuck was a big cowboy in his mid-forties from Houston whom I worked for back in the early Eighties. And for the first two months of working and living with Chuck he always wore a hat. Now, he liked hats - cowboy hats for going out, formal wear, baseball caps for casual wear, that sort of thing. But one night the emboldened Chuck came out of the hat box. And he took off his baseball cap at home to reveal he had the head of an American eagle.

Chuck you see was bald. And I was taken aback. I'd just assumed the hair I could see at the sides of his head reached all the way to his crown. And as Chuck took off his hat I could see he was stealing himself, nervous, but determined to make his own declaration of Houston Oilers hat independence. And I knew that this lovable but macho Texan hadn't loved hats enough to wear them in the house.

But it's not just good old boys like Chuck that struggle to declare a deep, longing desire to be at one with their hair again. Dr Pamela Wells of Goldsmith's College in London in 1995 produced a paper for the *British Journal of Psychology* which stated that bald people had markedly lower self-esteem than those with good hair covering.

She wrote; 'Far from being a laughing matter, male hair loss is associated with a marked decrease in psychological well-being. . . depression, neuroticism, introversion and a feeling of unattractiveness.'

David Thomas concurred. 'I know people who'll swear blind that going bald doesn't bother them.

'But I don't believe them, and nor does anyone on the hair replacement business.'

He goes on to reveals that Laurence Olivier, once lying desperately ill in hospital, 'with tubes everywhere', summoned his trichologist Philip Kingsley to his bedside and declared;

'I'm so worried about my hair. What can I do?'

But Dr Pamela's research confirmed what I'd always believed. It wasn't just old theatre luvvies who worried about hair loss. It was ordinary cowboys like Chuck. And ordinary Brits like me and David Thomas.

'The loss of one's hair is an infinitely depressing, confidence-sapping affair,' wrote the journalist.

'It bothers every slaphead, every chrome-dome, every baldy man. I find the idea of a wig, or even an Advanced Hair System (a weave) profoundly humiliating.

'But I'd kill to get my old hair back.'

There, Jim. Now do you believe me?

Big Alex, my painter and decorator pal certainly wasn't convinced transplants were a good idea. It wasn't acceptable he reckoned, for ordinary men to preen themselves. (Rather oddly, Big Alex wouldn't step outside the house unless he were completely co-ordinated; the socks *had* to match the tie.)

And when I told him the average cost of a hair transplant (around 6k) he didn't hold back on his thoughts.

"You're off your f****** head," he said, pun, I think, intended.

And so the mixed opinions continued. And to be honest, I was getting a little annoyed by the detractors. Some guys clearly felt that in yielding to cosmetic surgery I was invading women's territory. But I also think I represented a worry. What I was doing, I think, was holding up a mirror to some and offering a challenge, saying, 'Look, none of us look so hot at fifty. We could all do with a bit of work.'

What made the attacks all the more galling was the increased awareness that hair loss was a subject the pals in the pub – those with good hairlines that is - were overly keen to talk about. There was scarcely a Friday night went past when the subject of hair density didn't come up in conversation. And over the years I'd noticed that the reflections, comments on others' hair loss were all rather more frequent - and personal.

Women, on the other hand, would never say to each other; 'My those bingo wings are so well developed if you flap your arms you'll take off.' But men would gladly tell the same sex; 'You're getting a bit thin up there. Not long before you're polishing you're head right after you polish you're shoes.' They'd throw in old jokes; 'There is only one thing that stops hair from falling - the barber's floor.'

Why do men do it? It's because they are being primeval. It's about establishing superiority, it's about equating hair on head with manliness. And no hair with emasculation. The Hairfile contained this apposite story from *The Independent* in 1996.

'When Sean Lennoy discovered his wife was having an affair, a court heard last month, he decided to impose upon her lover the most humiliating punishment he could imagine. He held his rival down and rubbed Immac hair remover into his head.

'Unfortunately for Mr Lennoy, his rival re-grew stubble after four days. But the fact that this was held to be the ultimate embarrassment shows the degree to which hair loss among men is still seen as stigmatised.'

I came to understand that Hair Equals Power.

"Well, if you think you need to have a transplant . . . " said one of the dissenting voices.

"No, I don't *need* to. My thinning hair has never affected my social life. As far as I'm aware it's never ever stopped me getting a nice-looking girlfriend. I've never had to scrape the bottom of the barrel. But you've got a decent head of hair. So what's your excuse?"

Yes, I could be that waspish. And I gave up trying to convince the unconvincable.

Carry on regardless.

'For lack of a better term, they've
labelled me a sex symbol.
It's flattering and it should happen
to every bald, overweight guy.'

~ NYPD Blue star
Dennis Franz

12
The WW2 Transplant

AND so three months later, this morning in fact, I found myself standing outside the Farjo Clinic in the April sunshine feeling happily anxious, worriedly excited.

Well, it's not ever day you tick one of the largest personal boxes you've ever ticked in your life. And while for the past eleven hours or so I've remained happy and positive - and almost entirely relaxed having finally tackled the hair issue - there's still a little nagging concern.

I'm worried the final result won't look quite as I'd hoped. I'm worried that the new hair line doesn't somehow suit. I'm worried that it doesn't look as though it should be on my head.

Am I over-worrying now that it's all coming to an end? You bet. And I'm telling myself not to. However, I also know that I'm a bit on the fussy side. If I buy a shirt, for example, it has to be the right collar length, (no short, stumpy collars, no button downs (too schoolboy, or middle aged men trying to look cool) - the right material, (soft but not shiny cheap) exactly the right fit, shaped of course, no fold over cuff linked sleeves (unless it's a dress shirt) and certainly no Boris Johnson/Boris Becker contrasting white collars and stripes. You see what I'm saying? And a shirt is a whole lot more impersonal than a new head of hair.

Yes, I'm worrying. But not panicking. Not yet, anyway. And to be honest, a big part of me feels pleased with myself. I'm baldly going where few (Scots)men have gone before. I'm the Captain Kirk of hair restoration, set to discover this new world in which all (or most) men can have hair.

Sort of.

Just before coming down to Manchester, I realised I was slightly less of a pioneer than I had reckoned – just a recent chapter in an old story.

In 1939, Dr Okuda, a Japanese plastic surgeon actually carried out the world's first hair transplant on war victims, those with serious burns to the scalp. He extracted round plugs of hair-bearing skin and implanted them into slightly smaller round holes he made in the scarred or burnt areas. And although the results looked a little primitive his procedure worked.

Okuda was in fact the Godfather of modern transplant surgery. He had proved you could take hair from a 'permanent' place, i.e. the donor area - and move it around.

But although this was news the world (the balding world that is) was desperate to hear about, the success story didn't leave Japanese shores. Why? Well, a little political event called World War 2 was raging at the time. Hair transplanting wasn't a priority, unless you were one of the burns victims, and East-West science communications were non-existent.

It was more than 25 years later before the Western world was able to replicate Okuda's work.

But what if Okuda's work had become known to the

west? Would transplant techniques have raced forward?
Would Elton have been able to wear his own hair?

My thought is halted by the news jingle on radio. It's
now 6.30pm.

"We're not quite there yet," says Dr Farjo, whose talents
seem to include mind reading.

"But we're getting there. It's all looking good."

I'm in no rush though. And the longer the process takes
the more contented I feel. After all, if it had all been carried out rapidly I *would* have cause for worry. Time spent,
I reckon, equals effort plus professional concern. And I'm
still very much appreciative of the fact my future hair
density is being increased by the second.

Now, I'm laughing, and it's not entirely down to the
Chris Evans Show which is on in the background. I've
just thought of a lovely by-product of a successful hair
transplant.

Every FU placed means a FU to those in the pub who
teased those with less hair.

Every FU implanted means an FU to those who said I'd
end up looking like Elton, in spite of the fact I've never
worn ZOOM glasses, pink suits and been able to sing in
more than two octaves unless in serious pain.

And every FU that will eventually grow in my scalp
means a huge FU to those who said I'd be better spending
my money on a relaxing holiday and a sharp razor.

Well, I'll still be able to go on holiday next year - but
not have to rub factor 25 onto my scalp every morning.

"We won't be too long now," says Dr F, offering more
reassurance.

It's now 7pm and I'm still in no hurry to leave. Apart
from the fear of what my hairline will look like, my main

concern is for the hair doctor and his wife who've been standing longer than the Statue of Liberty.

But they're still going strong. And so is my imagination. I'm wondering if Evans is now deliberately playing lots of songs which have hair references in the lyrics?

What he starts off with is America's classic *Sister Golden Hair*. Then there's Sandy Thom's *Punkrocker* – 'with flowers in my hair.' Then Elvis is blasting out *Jailhouse Rock* and talking about fingers being ran through his hair.

Now I'm starting to think of songs with hair in the title; Jimmy Osmond's criminal classic *Long Haired Lover From Liverpool*. And there's *Hair* of course, the lead song from the musical. And *Bald* by The Darkness, (which, incidentally is the condition lead singer Justin Hawkins is headed unless he has some work done on his head.)

Okay, I admit it. I'm going a little OCD when it comes to the subject. Anyway, I'm blaming the Valium for leading me into the land of nonsense. But then one more band leaps into the head. Haircut 100.

Which leads me to another FU. It's to those hairdressers over the years, who never had hair line worries of their own, but seemed to take delight in informing me that I was going bald.

Right from my early twenties I'd be told that my hair was 'too thin' and my scalp 'too dry' and needed a special conditioner. Which, rather incredibly, they always seemed to have a bottle of, right on the shelf next to the till.

And you could never maintain that it was 'too expensive', even in times of student grants, because you just know they would ask the unanswerable question, 'What price do you put on your hair?'

Of course this 'special conditioner' – which had to be

used with the same-make shampoo – always cost twice as much as the haircut. And never seemed to work. The hair still collected around the plug hole after washing.

What this made me realise is that it's hugely important for a hair-thinning man to find a good hairdresser, someone with understanding, who comes to know your head better than the back of their own.

Leaving behind Uncle Chris in Canada and coming back to Britain to work in journalism meant living without a hair net, or rather a hair safety net, for a while. I'd try all sorts of hairdressers, from those in expensive salons to barber shops and had all sorts of set-backs. There were those who, because they'd cut hair for five years, reckoned they were practically a qualified trichologist.

And there were those who clearly didn't enjoy cutting thinning hair.

Okay, you've probably guessed that I've been permanently scarred by the Malky Kerr/Steve McQueen experience.

But you see, there is nothing more soul-destroying than sitting in the chair and having a stranger take a comb to your head, part your hair – delicately – and look down at your scalp because you just know at that moment they are thinking; 'Christ, there's not a lot going on here. I hope he doesn't ask me for anything too fanciful!'

What they invariably come out with is the stock cliché; 'And what would you like me to do for you today?'

Now, for some reason, male barbers - Trevor Sorbie and Uncle Chris and Stephen the Hamilton Hairdresser being exceptions - are rarely bald. They are clearly immune to DHT.

And what you really want to say to these hirsute hairdressers with their long, flowing frosted-tipped locks is

'I'll tell you what I'd like done. I'd like you to give me my hair back. Or, failing that, a haircut that doesn't accentuate my ever-increasing baldness. But since that's impossible, then just do your very best not to make me look like Uncle Fester.' But you don't say that. You say 'Just bring it in at the sides, tidy it up a little', or any of the mutterings that balding blokes use to reduce pressure on the beleaguered barber.

And then you sit back and watch them do their work. And you start to sweat as soon as the hair is washed because unlike at home where towel is applied to shower-wet hair immediately, you have to sit staring at your thread-thin, wet hair in the mirror.

Forever.

Now, when I had a haircut aged 17 in a unisex salon, or when Uncle Chris cut it, it wasn't a haircut at all, it was a hair *styling*.

But after the age of forty it was an endurance test. It was an exercise in staring cold, blunt reality in the face, your own face, looking in the mirror while a relative stranger with sharp scissors proceeds to lift strands of hair gingerly, cutting only the tiniest amount so's not to produce a shock result.

Sure, sometimes there would be a cute apprentice around who would give great head massage. But a haircut meant that every hair cut meant less covering available to the balding area. Every hair trimmed exposed more skin. Every hair that hit the floor was a sign that middle age was coming to get you with a baseball bat.

And even though hairdressers are, for the most part nice, sociable people, you know that they struggle at times to stay positive in the face of a face that's close to miserable.

They know that staring them in the face is a bloke who's watching his life, which is his hair, disappear before them.

The best that can be said about a visit to a hairdresser for the forty-plus, is that it's one of the few times you can sit down for half an hour and do nothing. (Sadly though, you can't close your eyes. You have to listen to the chat. Otherwise, your head will suffer.)

However, sometimes you find a hairdresser who manages to make you feel less anxious.

Like Sheenya.

For the past five years my ever-reducing hairline had been cut by Sheenya. And she was great because she was thin-hair sensitive. But even better, the ebullient blonde was always too pre-occupied in telling me about her love-life, her holiday adventures or the difficulties of bringing up twin teenage daughters on her own to overly bother about the worsening state of my head.

She could also give a very decent cut, as it happens. And in the past two years she even dropped the cost of the haircut by a fiver. She did it very subtly saying that she didn't like to charge me too much (£15) when what she really meant was that my hair loss had progressed to the point it could be cut in half the time.

Sheenya however had a smile on her face on hearing of my intention to have a transplant.

"What do you think, Sheenya? Should I go for it?"

"Well, you realise if you get more hair I'll have to put your haircut cost back up," she said, grinning.

"No, you can't, Sheenya. I'll have the same amount of hair on my head. It's just that it'll be moved around a bit."

She laughed. And I laughed. Yes. It was time for a new hair style.

But will it turn out to look the way I'd hoped? Gosh, I'm close to the point of discovery. The doctors Farjo are still pushing new life into my head. Pushing and dabbing with cotton. And now I'm looking at the clock on the wall. It's almost 7.30pm.

"We're done!" says Dr Farjo, sounding almost as jubilant as I feel.

Wow. It's over. After 12 hours in the chair I've survived a hair transplant. And I feel a tsunami-sized relief wash over me.

But what's it like? I desperately want to know.

Yet, I don't want to know. For varied reasons. I've enjoyed the hope that's come with the journey. Now, I don't know if I can cope if the result on my head is not the result I'd expected *in* my head.

And, if I'm not entirely happy, I don't want Dr Farjo to see a look of disappointment on my face. However, Bessam Farjo has already read what I'm thinking. He's probably seen this trepidation in clients a thousand times before.

And before I know what's happening he's standing in front of me holding a mirror in his hand.

It was really upsetting to lose my hair. I actually asked for a transplant at 18. It started to recede at the sides and I wasn't too worried about that but when it started to go in the middle it was hard.

~ Techo rock star **Gary Numan.**

13

A Tim Henman Hairline?

"WOULD you like to see what it looks like?" Dr Farjo is asking me.

And I'm terrified. I really am frozen with fear.

Not that I look like I've had a haircut from Sweeney Todd or that my bleeding, serrated and scarred head resembles a scene from *The Killing Fields*. I know that this is minor cosmetic surgery. No, the real worry is what if there's very little there, if it all looks bare as Mother Hubbard's Cupboard? Or what if the hairline looks weird, that it runs straight across my head like that of Frankenstein or Curly from *The Three Stooges*?

I know he drew a nice Napoleon Solo on my head during the initial consultation but this morning it was a bit too Tim Henman. And what about the scar line? I've left enough hair at the back to cover it over but . . .

I'm hesitating when I should be saying, with clear delight in my voice; "Oh, I can't wait to see my new hair."

And Dr Farjo picks up on this and looks a little, just a little, disappointed. And I pick up on the fact he's picked up on this. And I understand his disappointment. He's just spent over twelve hours creating a modern day miracle and I seem to be matter-of-fact. But I'm not. Far from it. I'm scared. Scared that it won't look like, one day, new hair will grow there happily and contentedly. Scared it will look patchy.

"No, I don't want to see what it looks like, Dr Farjo. I want to retain this feeling of quiet but contained optimism I'm enjoying. I want to leave this clinic and go out and have a nice dinner and sleep and dream about having flowing locks. What I don't want to do is look at my head and think 'Oh, God, no. The hairline is too squinty.'

But I'm not saying that to Dr Farjo. I'm thinking it. I'm thinking 'Not now, Dr Farjo. Let me face reality tomorrow'.

Yet, there is a large part of me that wants to see the result of this work right now. And above all, I don't want you to think me ungrateful. So what I really do say is "Yes, sure, let's have a look."

And now Dr Farjo is smiling. And he's holding the mirror up in front of me. And I'm taking the mirror from him and angling it so's I can see right onto my scalp.

And?

It looks fantastic! Incredible! Amazing! It's stunning. It's Steve McQueen. It's Cassidy. It's the dream come true.

It's the Kylie's bum of hair transplants.

The hairline doesn't run in a thick, straight line across my forehead. It isn't Timmy at all. It looks like the hairline of a 52 year-old man. It looks natural. It looks like me. Only better. With hair.

The implanted hairs that just 12 hours ago were living happily on the back of my head are tiny, having been shaved of course. But they're large enough to give the impression that this could be my field of dreams.

Yes, the scalp looks full. But not overly full. And I'm rejoicing. It's a wonderful feeling. For the first time in twenty years I now have a decent crop of hair on my head. Okay, it looks a little severe and odd because the hair at the side of my head is about an inch long while the stuff on top is shorter than Kylie. But overall, it still looks brilliant. I'm elated.

And Dr Farjo is looking pleased.

"I put in a few extra hairs," he says. "We managed to get more from the donor area than we had anticipated."

Wow! When we had the initial chat about what I could expect in terms of new hair Dr Farjo had anticipated on retrieving around 2,500 follicular units for transplant.

"I've implanted 3,200 units."

He adds, grinning; "I got a little carried away with myself."

And I'm so glad you did. (This is about the maximum amount of hairs that can be transplanted in any one session, although some people can get more.)

"Yes, it seems to have come out very well," says Dr Farjo.

And I still have the mirror in my hand. And I'm still looking at all those little hairs in wonder. I know how they came to be there. But I still can't believe it.

God, I wish Uncle Chris were around to see it.

Of the 3,200 follicular unit grafts implanted in my head, I learned later that of these, 480 were single hair units, 2333 were two hair units and 387 were made up of three and four hair units. That's why it looks natural. The single units are used mostly at the front to give a hairline. But the spacing is important, it has to look slightly imperfect in order to give a close to perfect appearance.

What matters though is that the top of my head has now around 6,300 hairs. And they will all fall out of course, as the hair breaks off from the follicle. But each will be set to make their re-appearance on my head just about the time the leaves will start to fall from the trees.

"The back of your head will be a little sore for a few days," says Dr Farjo.

"And your scalp will be numb for a while because of the pressure on the nerve ends. But the feeling will come back soon."

Well, I'm sure it will. But for the moment all I'm thinking about is the future, that these little slivers of hair will grow into long shafts.

And now I'm leaving the big seat, making my way into the post-operative room. I'm still a little woozy from the Valium, but not overly so.

And I'm being offered the choice of a baseball cap or a woolly hat, for a cover up. The scalp is close to purple in colour.

And while I think it looks wonderful - I'm focusing on the short shafts rather than the pigmentation - others may think it looks odd.

"I'll take the baseball cap, thanks."

The cap is placed rather gingerly on my head. And the back of my scalp feels a little tender. But that doesn't matter. For the next twenty minutes Dr Farjo gives me my post-op instructions and a sheet of *Do's* and *Don'ts*; *Sleep With Several Pillows Under Your Head, Don't Sunbathe And Let Your Scalp Burn, Be Careful Not To Bump Your Head. Do Not Bend Over To The Floor Over The Next Two Days*, that sort of thing.

He also hands me a little toilet bag which contains special shampoo, conditioner and antiseptic spray and painkillers. I'm set. Ready to leave.

"Would you like a lift round to the hotel?" says Dr Farjo.

"I'm going past that way."

By this time the Blonde has given up waiting for me. She'd been in the clinic and gone back to the hotel.

"Thanks, that would be great."

Hopefully, I thanked Dr Farjo enough as I left the clinic and headed for Chinatown with the Blonde for a celebration dinner.

I say hopefully, because I felt so full of joy that all I could think about was this fantastic new hair line that will one day be mine for keeps.

****

FIVE minutes later I'm at the Arora Hotel. It's nice and friendly. I meet the Blonde and she can't wait to have a peek under my cap.

"It looks great!" she says with real enthusiasm.

"Your scalp looks a bit sore but you can see all the little hairs. It will look fantastic."

Ten minutes later we're in a Chinese restaurant. I'm quite hungry, which is a sign that I'm not feeling any ill-effects of the procedure.

I've a feeling I'm being stared at however by one or two people and that's because I am. I'm wearing a baseball cap indoors and it's no longer trendy. But little do the diners know the blue cap is concealing a purple head and the results of 12 hours of scalp-scraping and space-filling.

A couple of hours later, I'm ready to sleep. The t-shirt is a little awkward to pull over my head and I need assistance to take it off (Yes, I should have followed the guidelines and worn a shirt with buttons down the front).

And the idea of having several pillows propping up my head doesn't fill me with glee. Usually I have a single pillow, which is as flat as the first day back at work after a holiday. But I persevere. Dr Farjo's supplied toilet bag of post-op aids came with a little towel which is to be placed under the head in case of some night-time bleeding and I do that. Gosh, will I sleep? My mind is racing. However the events of the day and the two Cocodamol pills must have conspired to make sure I slept pretty well.

The next thing I know it's morning. And I'm looking at the little towel and there isn't a blood mark on it. Great. No problems with the stitches or anything. What does the head feel like? Tight. And a bit numb. And I'm touching the scalp very gingerly with the tip of my finger but I don't feel anything. Literally. I really don't have much sensation in the scalp. And that's what I was told it would be like.

And now I'm looking in the mirror. I don't look fantastic to be honest. The long hair at the sides looks a bit sticky and messy, and it contrasts with the top. The scalp is now very purple-looking; not quite *Black Night* deep purple but nor is it Sindy Doll pink. But I take a positive from this; the darker scalp colour gives the illusion of having more hair.

I'm having a little bit of bother with my clean t-shirt though. I need the Blonde's help to get it over my head without making contact with my head. Yes, I know I really should have brought a shirt to wear instead but that would have been too sensible.

After breakfast I'm back in the clinic. Dr Farjo knew I was staying overnight and asked me to pop in for a quick look. We chat about the Chinese restaurant – an excellent recommendation – and he looks at my scalp.

"It's fine," he says. "We'll give it a quick wash."

"Is that not a bit soon? Won't it cause the hair follicles

to fall out?" He's looking at me and wondering if I'm joking, half-serious or daft. But he says nothing, probably realising that I'm a mix of all three.

Plus, a little vulnerable.

We get to chatting. I tell him I'm taking today and tomorrow (Thursday and Friday) off work and heading back on Monday.

He points out that lots of men who have the transplants arrange a holiday directly afterwards. Usually in the Greek islands for some reason.

Perhaps such a vanity project has to be celebrated in a culture where male vanity is not considered a negative trait? Who knows.

But the holiday means they can go off and relax and let the head heal. And it also means there is less chance of having to explain the purple head or why there's a baseball cap attached to the top of their body where there's never been one before.

It makes sense. And I thought perhaps I should have thought about that. What the hell, it's done now.

The shampoo is over and I don't feel much up top except a lot cleaner. Then Dr Farjo takes a series of photographs.

Ten minutes later, I'm chatting to Mick. There's now a shared experience between us, we've both gone through a transplant, and he's one of the few people who knows what's going on in my head at the moment.

We get to chatting about the re-growing of my original hair, i.e. the little hair I had left on my scalp and I tell Mick it would be nice to hang onto that, to have it alongside the new hair that will grow.

"Well, the new hair will grow in four to five months

time," says Mick. "But your old hair will continue to fall out."

Unless?

At this point I recall that Dr Farjo, during my original consultation, suggested I could try the Finasteride. And I recall that Finasteride, known more commonly as Propecia or Proscar, is said to slow hair loss in 83 per cent of men - and has even led to re-growth in 66 per cent of men.

I think hard. And I recall that Spencer Kobran had had great results with Proscar.

'Within twelve months, ninety-five percent of my hair was actually growing again. It was still a little thinner than it had been before the onset of male pattern baldness, but I was no longer concerned with losing my hair and the unwanted change in my appearance.'

And Kobren, like Mick, had had no adverse side effects, sexual or otherwise.

Oh, well. Why not? And I buy the Finasteride. I can justify the outlay. Keep the hair that I had, perhaps make it thicker.

Yes, I know my pal's pal took it and it left him short of solid oak furniture in the bedroom department. But if that happens I can always stop.

There. Done. And off home, with a smile of completion, of happy expectation on my face.

Yet, I can't help but wonder what the reaction to my newly-styled head will be.

Part 2

14

The Hairgod's Hair

IT'S Day Two PT (post transplant) and Friday night. I'm in the pub with my pal, Ian, and wearing the baseball cap. I feel a bit self-conscious, not because I'm hiding the fact I've had a hair transplant, but because middle-aged men who wear baseball caps indoors are trying that wee bit too hard to look cool.

I don't *have* to cover the scalp; I'm not fearful of bumping. And the only thing likely to drop on my head is the odd heavy stare. Yet, at the same time I'm not ready to go public. After all the scalp is still the colour of a nice Merlot, the transplant just a bristle and I have longer hair on the sides.

In short, I need to wait until I get a short(er) back and sides and less of a red grape colour on the head before I reveal it to the world.

Ian is curious about how it all went.

"Is the head painful? Are you glad it's all over?"

"No, the head is not painful. It feels a bit tender at the back but the top is still numb-ish. And tight."

Now I remember why it's important that Dr Farjo said I had a nice elastic scalp. When you lose half and inch of it all round there is less of it available to fit over your head.

But the skin will stretch I'm told. And it has, to a degree. Yet, I still feel like I'm wearing my wee sister's bathing cap.

"So how long will it be before you've got more hair on your head than a horse? What you've got at the moment looks great."

"Ah, you see there's the thing. The transplant hair that you see before you, or at least had a swatch at before we came in here, will fall out in the next few days.

"And it will be four or five months before it grows back in."

"That's not such a long time to wait."

"No, but I feel like a 12 year-old who's been given a brand new, shiny ten-speed racer with Shimano gears to race around in for a week. Then your mum tells you you can't ride it again until September."

"Yes, but that bike will be yours. And you'll love it all the more for having had to wait a while to ride it."

And he's right. I feel almost smug. I'm looking around the bar and knowing that the word will have spread by now that the reason my head is wearing a blue Kickers baseball cap is because I've had work done.

And I know that there will be a real curiosity about it - and some snorts of derision. But I know there will come a time when it will grow back.

It will grow. Won't it?

Come to think of it, is there a guarantee it will grow back? Yes, I remember now. I had this conversation with Mick during the first phone call.

"We guarantee 90-95 per cent success rates," said Mick.

"What does that mean, Mick. That for five to 10 per

cent of men the procedure doesn't work at all? Or do you guarantee that 90-95 per cent of the hair transplanted into clients heads will actually grow?"

"Yes, the latter. Most of the hair will grow effectively. And if there is a visible area in which it doesn't, Dr Farjo will sort it."

"With a further transplant?"

"Yes, it will be fixed. But I have to say cases where people aren't completely satisfied are rare. I can't recall any in fact."

Great. There you are. It will grow. So stop worrying.

"Stop worrying," says Ian, reading my concern. "You kicked back against the forces of nature and you've won."

And we laugh at how cruel and capricious nature can be. Those who get the short end of the genetic stick will find their male hormones starting to take away the hair on their heads just when they're commanding other body hair to become long and coarse. And the same hormonal attack that produces testosterone which develops into DHT can also react with the oil producing glands to create acne.

Can you imagine it? Going bald as a teenager and getting acne? It made me think back to poor Sparky. But at least his acne also disappeared.

"Was your dad bald?" asks Ian.

"No, he wasn't. He had hair like Elvis. And, sadly, lived about the same length of time for roughly the same reasons. But even if your father has a great hair line, that doesn't mean you will enjoy great hair."

"I thought baldness was hereditary."

"Well, it is sort of. I've been reading up on this and to be a candidate for baldness a man simply has to have a genetic predisposition toward it. This is possible if anyone in his family, on either side, has ever been bald.

"Then if a bloke has the normal complement of male hormones to carry out the genetic code's instructions, it's just a matter of time."

Ian, who has a decent head of hair, absorbs this information. Now, he may just be humouring me, or perhaps he is genuinely interested.

He doesn't seem bored at all when I quote the American gene pool stats that show the percentage of bald men runs just about parallel with age: 25 per cent of 25-year-olds, 50 per cent of 50-year-olds, 75 per cent of 70 year-olds.

He even laughs when I tell him of a story I had stored in the Hairfile, about the anatomy professor from Howard University who in 1965 claimed that baldness was caused by great intelligence.

This Government-funded halfwit tried to prove that the brain grew larger in smart men, stretching the scalp across the head until it was too tight to hang onto the hair.

Now, those thinning liked to buy into that notion. And I'd bet that this professor wasn't a hirsute handsome man with a regular sized head at all.

From nutty professors we leapt to the subject of baldness and virility. You know how bald guys are always claiming they are more virile? Well it's a myth. Who says? Well, Estelle Ramey, Georgetown University medical school physiology professor and an expert on hormonal effects, does.

The ability to get an erection and sustain it is much more a function of the nervous system than the hormones. 'The nervous system's role is so powerful, in fact, that a sexually active man can be castrated and, even without hormone replacement, remain sexually potent for a year,' she writes.

"Let's hope that we never put the theory to the test," says Ian.

But matters of genetic predisposition don't have to bother me any longer. At least, not as far as hair goes.

I hope.

＊＊＊＊＊＊＊＊＊＊＊＊

IT'S Saturday and three days after the transplant. And a lot has happened to my head since. It's been washed three times now. With Aussie Shampoo. Ph balanced. Just to be safe. And that in itself is a bit of a chore. The post PT instruction notes said not to rub shampoo directly onto the scalp, but to apply it first to a small towel, then place towel on head and let the shower fall on towel.

This is to prevent the head taking a battering, and perhaps disrupt the new follicles. And the rinsing process is the same. All in all, it adds an extra ten minutes to the shower time, but . . . needs must.

The head hasn't been sore, there's been no bleeding or anything drastic like that and no signs of infection at all. But it's still numb on top, and it feels rather tight. And it has been a little itchy at the back. However, each morning and night I've been spraying the top and back with Dr F's magic antiseptic spray and it's cooling and soothing, and that seems to do the trick. The top of my head however has now become plum-coloured. And the little hair shafts are still there. But I need to have a haircut. It's too long at the sides. The contrast with the top is so great and I look like John Malkovich with a scalp courtesy of the Dulux *Warm Bedroom Colours* range.

And I wish I'd perhaps arranged a holiday straight after transplant after all. As it is, I'm set to go back to work on Monday. Think. I need a haircut. But I can't count on Sheenya. The salon she works in has closed up for good and she's decided to take a sabbatical from hair snipping and colouring and spend time with her cute but troublesome 14 year-old blonde twins, lest they turn into Mary-Kate and Ashley Olsen with ASBOS.

I feel vulnerable. I need a haircut. Verisimilitude is called for. But I haven't been to another hairdresser for years. And I certainly don't feel comfortable about walking into a stranger's salon, taking off the baseball cap and showing them my purple head, if you pardon the expression.

I can't be bothered talking to a perfect stranger, or even a slightly imperfect one, all about the hair transplant process, that the hair they see before them on top of my head would soon be gone, but would come back etc, etc.

I can't bear the thought of a 19 year-old saying to me; 'Going anywhere nice for your holidays? Going anywhere special tonight? Didn't Elton have a dodgy hair transplant once?' in consecutive sentences.

Yet, I need to have something done. I don't want to go back to work on Monday wearing a hat, sitting there in a newspaper office looking like Joe Di Maggio in a suit. No thank you. Thankfully, the Blonde comes up with a solution. She knows a young-ish hairdresser in the village where we live, Vinnie, and calls him and tells him of my little dilemma. Vinnie suggests I come down to the salon just after it closes and he will see what can be done. And that's what I do. Three hours later I'm sitting in Vinnie's red chair.

"I've never seen a hair transplant before," he says, looking down at my head and then gently taking a peek at the scar line beneath my hair at the back at the sides.

"You know, the scar doesn't look bad at all. And your scalp seems fine. Just a bit off-colour."

'Off-colour'. Sensitivity. I like that.

And he is genuinely interested in the process; the hair re-growth period, the division of the follicles, the placing.

"Where does the new hair come from? Do they take it from your leg?" (Well, it seems a sensible enough question, given that surgeons often turn to the leg or the backside for spare body bits.)

And he studies the layout on my head like a serious punter studies the racing form on a Saturday morning.

"It all looks really natural," he enthuses.

"I think you'll get a good result here."

Just then Vinnie's mobile rings. It's his girlfriend, sorting out their Saturday night plans. And while he chats I pick up a glossy magazine to browse through. And there on the cover is the Hairgod himself.

David Cassidy.

It's a recent pic. And I find myself looking closer at the star who was once the most famous man in the world, with songs that made young girls cry and a great hair covering that young men (like me) tried to copy.

David Cassidy's still got a lot of hair. And nowadays he combs it backwards. But my eyes are drawn to the hairline. It seems *very* specific. All those little frontline hairs seemed to be lined up in perfect formation like a Roman legion.

Could they be relatively new to that part of his head? Mmm. I'm wondering if the American star has had a little HT work done.

Does David Cassidy have David Cassidy hair these days? And I make a mental note to steer that into the conversation the next time I interview him. But at the same time I'm laughing gently at the notion that perhaps even the Hairgods aren't any more immune to hair loss than the rest of us.

And now Vinnie is catching the grin on my face, seeing me smiling, no doubt thinking the delight has come from looking at myself in the mirror for three minutes.

No matter.

He's now taking his clippers to the sides. Gently. And he's good. I don't feel a thing. And at the back where the scar was a little more sensitive he uses his scissors to get the longer hair as short as possible and closer to the length on top. And it works. It looks a whole lot better.

Sorted. For a tenner. Brilliant.

Three hours later however and settling for a night in watching TV I feel some discomfort, and not just because I've had to miss out on my mighty Saturday afternoon tennis match with my pal Stephen. (Rule 5 of the Post-Op Instructions said; *No strenuous physical activity for one week after surgery; e.g, sex, jogging, sport, gym.*)

No, it's awkward to lean my head back in the sofa and relax because after ten minutes pressure or so the back of my head feels a little tender, or itchy. But, overall, it's nothing to bother about. And sleep comes easily, thanks to taking a Cocodamol before dropping off.

IT'S now Sunday. And feeling fine I decide to fly in the

face of Dr F's instructions and go out on my bike. Slowly, though. Just to get the blood flowing. But Dr Farjo's instructions are on the money. Even the slow movement of morning cycling makes me feel a queasy and I resolve to wait a few more days before hitting the saddle again.

The Blonde didn't think I should be doing any exercise at all.

"You're off your head," she rebuked.

The afternoon produces another test. My mother checks out the transplant, and all the little hairs, and thinks it looks 'great'.

And I think her delight is genuine, even though I know if I'd had the top of my scalp dyed emerald green my mother would still have said it looked great.

"Does that mean you'll have real hair again?" she quizzes.

"Real as you can get," I said.

"That's good. You can see already it makes such a difference."

Her tone suggested she'd had some concerns about my disappearing hairline. She'd spoken in the past about how her brother, Alex, 'didn't suit' having gone bald.

Another hair flashback.

I remember once, I was about thirteen at the time, she actually took me to the doctors because she was worried about my hair. 'He's worried about his hair, doctor,' she said to the elderly old gent, which wasn't true at all.

I thought my hair was fine. (My early Malky experience had been forgotten). She must have felt that it was too fine. But now I remember feeling less than fine that she had reckoned I needed medical assistance.

Dr Van Collier was however a reassuring sort. Old

school. And he prescribed something called Polytar Shampoo. I don't know what it was supposed to do but I do recall that it smelled like melted wellies that had been worn for six years by an aged building site labourer with chronic athlete's foot.

And I do recall washing my pre-David Cassidy, still short, hair - still being cut by Malky Kerr - with this brown bottle of brown liquid for quite some months, perhaps even a couple of years, before having the bottle to return to regulation Vosene or whatever was around the bathroom.

Did the Polytar make any difference? Not that I can remember, except making my head smell funny. And I do recall picking up a couple of comments from less-than-sensitive schoolmates about nit shampoo and the like.

Tomorrow however, it's comments from workmates I'm a little concerned about. It will be my first day back. And while there are some who know I've had a couple of days off to get new hair, 'A procedure', as Helen on the news desk described it, there are others who don't have a clue.

Will I have the mickey ripped right out of me? Well, that's what I'm expecting.

But I've got a plan.

'When others kid me about being bald, I simply tell them that the way I figure it, the good Lord only gave men so many hormones, and if others want to waste theirs on growing hair, that's up to them.'

~ Astronaut **John Glenn.**

15

Cornflake Head

NEWSPAPER journalists are not renowned for their great sensitivity. I *knew* I was in for a hard time today when I walked into the office.

That's why I wore a wig.

No, I didn't go out and spend a few hundred quid to take the bare look off my head and try to pretend to people that I actually had a good head of hair. I wore a party shop wig that cost me seven quid, which I'd bought to wear to a Sixties fancy dress party a few years ago. And although it was made out of genuine nylon, it didn't look *that* bad at the time. It didn't look real of course, but I'd cut it and styled it to fit, (those years spent living with a hairdresser uncle weren't wasted at all), and from a distance it looked a little Davy Jones of the Monkees c1967.

But what was fascinating was the reaction I got in the office. The Editor laughed immediately, no doubt seeing that I was taking the mickey out of myself. Yet, over at the sports desk I noticed there was some serious discussion going on.

After a few minutes football reporter Ronnie called me over.

"What are you doing?" he said.

"What do you mean, Ronnie?"

"Well . . ." he stuttered . . . "the hair."

"What about the hair?" I asked, keeping a seriously straight face.

"It's not . . . real, mate."

"No, Ronnie. I've had a hair transplant."

"Have you f***! It's, it's . . . a wig."

"No, I've had a hair transplant."

Now, at this point all of the sports desk became engrossed in this conversation. They, like Ronnie, didn't know about the HT. They assumed I'd given up the bald look and gone out that weekend and bought myself a highland jig.

And a very bad one at that.

Ronnie was worried for me. Big time. And now the rest of the office, about a hundred journos, were listening in.

"Are you sure . . . you know what you're doing," said Ronnie, his voice betraying his concern for my sanity.

"Yes, I've had a hair transplant, Ronnie."

And he dipped his own head, in deep worry. And at that point I pulled off the wig to reveal the almost bald purple head with the little shafts of hair. And Ronnie's face lit up with relief.

"You're a complete bastard," he said. Affectionately.

From that point on the rest of the office went about their business, writing Kid Courage stories, or football reports or TV reviews. My hair story was no longer news. And that was exactly what I wanted. (For the moment at least.)

Interestingly, my head didn't bother me at all during the course of the day. Not in a physical sense. Not only was there no pain at all, there was no irritation.

Right now however I'm at home, trying to relax and watch TV. And it's a little awkward when I try to put my head back on the sofa. The donor area feels a little tender. And it's also itchy. There's a temptation to scratch. But I console myself with the thought that it's not desperate, not like when I had chicken pox, or the time I broke my tibia and had a full length plaster for six months - and the top of my foot became itchy and I used a wire coat hanger to scratch it and nearly ripped my shin open. No, this is easier to deal with. And a little spray of Dr Farjo's anti-septic does the trick.

FIVE days later and the head is settling nicely. Sarah at the next desk has taken to taking photos of my scalp every morning on her phone, 'so's we can see how it's coming along'. But for the most part people ignore my new top.

During the next few days however friends such as Lesley call to hear how it has all gone. I tell her that it went well and that you can see the transplanted hairs, but in a few days they will fall out and not re-grow for another three months at least.

She offers words of comfort, in her own inimitable black-humoured cold-as-death manner only a journalist could conjure up.

"Think of these hairs as baby teeth," she says, laughing wickedly.

"They'll fall out - but then you'll get your real teeth. And no one can every call you an ugly wee gap-toothed child again."

Strangely, I'm comforted by her comments.

IT'S ten days after HT. Saturday morning and the purple head has gone. It's not quite it's natural pink colour yet, but it's getting closer. It looks a bit crusty thanks to the little scabs that have formed. The top of my head looks like someone has crushed up cornflakes and glued them to my scalp. Most people wouldn't notice them though. And to be honest they don't look that bad. I did bend down to pick up my train ticket yesterday and the schoolboy standing next to me had a quizzical look on his face when I looked up. But beyond that there hasn't been a mention of the effect at work.

I don't get 'Hello Cornflake Head' when I walk into the office in the morning. Some of the scabs have even started to fall off. The trick is to resist the urge to pick them off. But I have developed the habit of touching my head religiously. It's as if I'm checking that all is well with that part of the world.

The problem is that as the scabs fall out, the little transplanted hair shafts fall to earth, or more likely the bottom of my shower tray, right along with them. Oh well. At least the original hair, or what was left of it, is already growing back in.

Isn't nature wonderful.

But it's time to move on. And today is the day Dr Farjo suggested I could have my stitches removed. That's a blessing because my head has been feeling a little tight. It will be nice to have them all gone. Yet, I don't know if the scarring has healed sufficiently. I don't go to the local surgery however and ask the nurse to remove them. Instead, my guitar-playing pal Jim offers to come round my house and take them out. This isn't as wild an idea as you may think. Jim may be cool hand with a Fender Stratocaster but he is also a top consultant. And he comes round, surveys the stitching - and gives it top marks.

"This is excellent work," he says.

"The doctor who's stitched your head certainly knows what he's doing. He's used the trichophytic stitching and it really works. The scar line looks fantastic."

Trichophytic closure entails trimming one edge of the cut prior to closure. When the opposing edge of the cut is joined to the trimmed edge it results in hairs from the trimmed edge growing through the resulting scar - effectively camouflaging its appearance. It takes way longer than regular stitching, but the results are there not to be seen.

"I won't take all the stitches out," says Jim.

"It will be uncomfortable. What we'll do is just let them dissolve. But I'll take a couple of the bigger ones out at the side of your head, where they are knotted, and that will release the tension."

And with a deft touch, Jim cuts away the plastic string that has made sleep a little uncomfortable - yet has played its part in holding my head together.

Instantly, I feel the pressure on my head is released. The tightness is gone, like someone letting the air out of a match ball that's been over-inflated.

Ah. Relief.

Jim is pleased too. Not just at the work done. After the de-stitching business he discovers I've got a David Bowie songbook from the Seventies and he borrows it with the intent of scanning in all the chords of the likes of *Suffragette City* and *Starman*.

Now, all I have to think about is my return to the white-hot heat of the tennis court. I'm playing Stephen this afternoon. He's twelve years younger and almost as industrious as Nadal.

Six hours later and I'm reflecting that the return to the tennis arena was premature. I couldn't hit the ball for the life of me. Normally the games with Stephen are fairly close but today my opponent beats me senseless. Somehow, my body was telling me that I shouldn't have been on the tennis court. Not yet, anyway. Annihilated. In three straight sets.

I don't know whether I was thinking about the blood rushing to my head or the effects of the procedure had had an effect. Or perhaps it was just the lack of any real exercise for ten days.

There was an interesting exchange however at the tennis club with another sometime partner, Paul, whom I bumped into just before going on court.

"Haven't seen you about," said Paul.

"Nope. Been in Manchester. Had a hair transplant."

"Eh?"

"Yes. Wanted to have it done for a while."

"A hair transplant? Is that not really vain?"

"Don't know, Paul. Is it really vain, or just mildly vain? I can never work it out."

"Let's see what it looks like."

And Paul, who doesn't have a lot of hair on his head, and is about ten years younger, had a good look at my scalp.

"I can see all the wee hairs. Will they grow?"

"First they'll fall out. Then they'll grow in. By Christmas I'll be wearing a John McEnroe headband to stop the hair falling into my eyes."

Now, Paul didn't laugh. He paused for a moment. And he deliberated. I could see a curiosity in his eyes.

"How does it work?" he said. And so I explained the process, taking the hair from the donor site etc.

Then he thought for a moment before asking; "Do you think a hair transplant would work for me?"

"I don't know, Paul. Depends upon how much hair you've got at the back of your head. Let's see."

And so from being accusatory two minutes beforehand, Paul's mind was now racing with the possibility – for the very first time in his existence – that he didn't have to be bald.

I could see that single thought was a little staggering to him.

"What does it cost," he said, coming back to Earth a little.

"Depends on how much hair you want/can have," I said. And so he trooped off to play, a little confused, but with the light of possibility switched on in his shiny head, a man released from the prison of his own limited imagination.

Clearly, issues of vanity had been conquered by possibility.

I tell my son that don't have
any hair because I gave it to
him when he was born, so he
actualy still believes that.
He's five years old.'

~ **Andre Agassi**

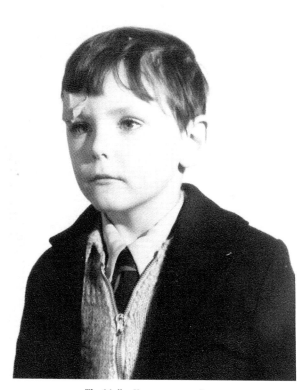

The Malky Kerr crew cut days.

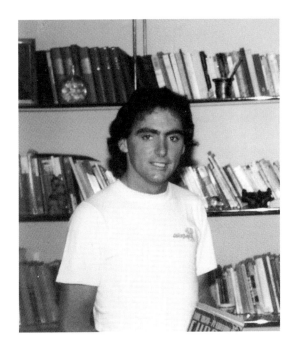

David Cassidy hair days.

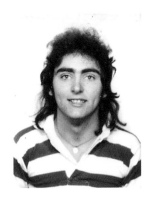
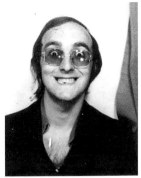

Sparky, fast losing it.

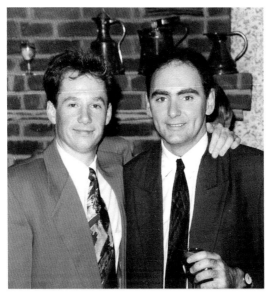

Me and Colin in 1993. The hair is thinning.

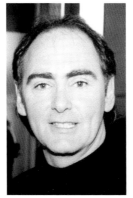

Really starting to thin out 1996.
Time to consider options.

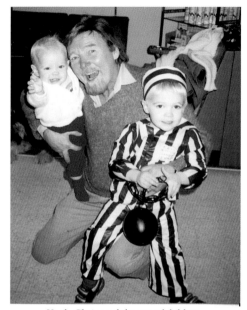

Uncle Chris and the grandchildren.

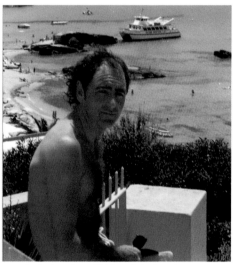

*At the beach in 2005 and the hair has gone
out with the tide.*

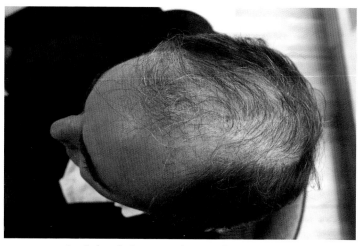

Just before the hair transplant. Really is time to act.

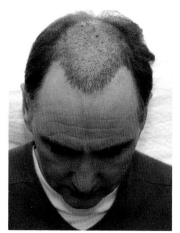

Just after the hair transplant.
It looks sore but . . .

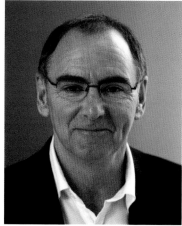

Three months later, new hair is
on the way.

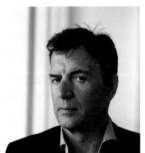

*Duncan Bannatyne (Pic credit:
Evening Times)*

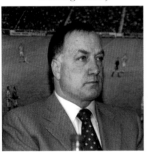

*Dick Advocaat
(Pic credit: Evening Times)*

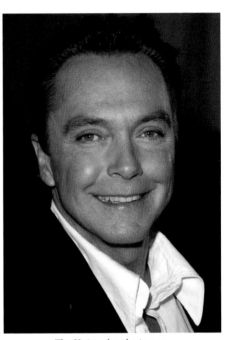

The Hairgod as he is now.

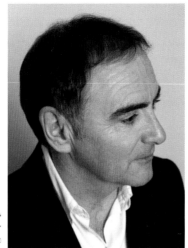

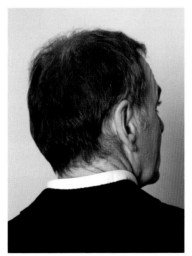

© BAM Photography.

The final results

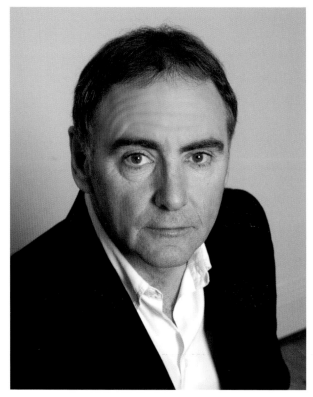

Not quite David Cassidy c1973. But it's still growing.

16
The Grave Digger Look

TWO weeks PT and the scalp is fine, the scabs are all but gone and people at work don't give me a second glance - my story is now chip paper in their heads. And I've come to terms with the fact the little shafts of transplanted hair have also all but gone.

Sort of.

I'm now as close to being as bald as I was as a new-born baby.

But I've comforted myself somewhat with the thought at least some of the old hair is making a comeback; I can feel the little shoots of recovery. And the new hair will appear. At some point. Yet, I had a strange sensation this morning when |I got caught in the rain. For the first time, I felt the water plinking onto my coverless head. It was an odd feeling and I can't say I found it pleasant at all. I began to think about Sacha Distel's delight while singing *Rain Drops Keep Falling On My Head* and getting annoyed because the Frenchman had a hairline as strong as the Eiffel Tower.

However, that odd experience was nothing compared to the one I suffered in the office. Around 10am when I at-

tacked my toast and banana breakfast I found myself
chewing on a piece of plastic, a bit of plastic knife or
something.

Yet, when I pulled it from my mouth the 'plastic' wasn't.
It was a tooth. My tooth. My broken front tooth.

"Aargh!" I screamed. And the office looked around. This
was a real trauma. A genuine frightener. Why would I be
eating toast when seconds later I'm eating one of my
most
important molars? Teeth just don't break off. It's all very
well hairs falling out. That's down to genetics and the evil
DHT, as we know. But teeth? Scary business.

At the speed of light, I called the dentist. And Alistair,
although always busy because he likes to work mornings
and then head for the golf/garden/snooker, said he would
sort me out.

Forty minutes later I'm walking into his surgery. And
he's looking at me and doesn't seem worried about the
tooth at all. He seems more concerned about what has
been happening to my head.

"What kind of shriking (his version of a sweary word)
haircut is that?" he demands, laughing.

"A short one?"

"Short? It's frightening!"

"Well, Alistair, I've had a hair transplant."

"Have you hell..."

"No, honestly. When I lay down in that chair you'll see
the stitches.'

Now, at this point he's realises I'm not joking. And he
looks a wee bit uncomfortable. And he feels that he's
made *me* feel uncomfortable. So I help him out a bit.

"Look, I know what you're thinking; if this is an example

of a hair transplant it's not a very good one."

"Yes," he grins, breathing a sigh of relief.

"Ah, but here's the thing. This is not how it will look in four months time. It has yet to grow in."

"So you'll have real hair? Growing? And that's not the finished result."

"God, I hope not!"

"Great. Well, good for you."

That sorted, he's examining my tooth - which I'd brought with me, and it has had a hairline crack, caused by a filling from years before.

Thank goodness. And now he's poking around a bit with his little steel stick, drilling a little, pulling and hauling a bit. And now he's glueing the broken tooth back in.

"Will it last?" I ask.

"I don't know. I've glued one broken tooth back in that's still there years on and yet another only lasted a few weeks. But it's worth a go."

It is. And on the train back to the office the tooth issue gives me something to chew over. I realise that my hair transplant experience had been a lot less traumatic than a visit to the dentist. I'm not overly terrified of dentists, and Alistair is as skilled as they come, but as soon as someone starts scratching around with what look like instruments of medieval torture I want to be out of there. As soon as that drill whines and you start to smell burning and taste pieces of your own bone I grip the arms of those big chairs for all they are worth.

No, sir. Give me a day on the HT clinic chair with a DVD to watch any time. But the trip to the dentist also provided me with a moment of clarity. It made me realise that 150 years ago, without dentists and their wonderful glue right now I'd look like a Dickensian grave-digger.

Of course, I didn't *have* to have my tooth fixed; it didn't hurt or anything and I could still manage to chew food. But the world from that point onwards would have judged me, viewed me as a moron/deviant/hillbilly. And my vanity/personal pride demanded I get the tooth repaired.

So what's the difference in having a hair transplant? Balding, and toothlessness, after all, makes people look older and less attractive. A report in the British Medical Journal stated that 'Baldness can add ten years to a person's appearance.'

There. Confirmed. Now, the next time a bloke suggests I'm a bit vain for having had the HT, can I simply enquire how much dental work he's had done?

There's also an argument that having less hair can also be career threatening. Radio and television presenter Johnny Vaughn agrees. Or at least he did back in the early Nineties when I interviewed him during his TV *Moviewatch* stint.

Johnny was a great interview subject, full of high octane conversation and revealing for the first time how he'd once been a coke dealer and ended up in pokey. But he also made another very honest comment.

I mentioned I thought he had a really good career ahead of him and he threw in a telling caveat.

'If I can keep my hair,' he said. 'It's getting a bit thin on top. And you can't be a bald and be a presenter. It just doesn't work.'

Perhaps that's why Johnny seems to work mostly on radio these days. Judging by recent photos of a shaved head it seems he hasn't gone down the road of hair addition. And I have to be honest, the career aspect played a part in my decision to have the transplant.

Just a few weeks before the procedure I took off for the day to an adventure course in the Highlands, to climb trees, to swing on ropes, to slide on high wires. It was a break from writing about actors and television and even though the falling rain was of Biblical proportions it was good fun.

But the next day as I looked at the story as it was set to appear in the paper I had one of those jolts that hit me to the core. The central pic in the story was of me swinging on a rope. But as it was taken, and I was smiling for the camera, my woolly hat fell off. I looked completely, utterly, bald. Hairless. I looked like a bloke in his sixties. I looked like someone who shouldn't be out swinging on trees.

And here's where the vanity really kicked in; I had the features ed pull the pic and substitute it with one – a poorer picture – in which I'm wearing the hat. Yes, I let vanity get in the way of a good double page spread.
I didn't want readers to see me as I really am. Bald.

And I'm bald right now, but at least there's the comfort in knowing I won't be for too much longer.

And thankfully, pals manage to help me see the funny side of the situation. Such as Ford. This afternoon he calls to talk about a writing idea and during the chat he asks a very odd, seemingly tangential, question.

"Listen, did you realise you have so much in common with Felix Fritzel?"

"No."

And I could sense a gag coming on but I was already curious. Felix Fritzel is the deranged Austrian who kept his daughter in a dungeon and used her as sex slave.

"So, Ford, what have I any common with this lunatic?"

"You've both had hair transplants!" he announces.

"It's a rather unfortunate comparison, don't you think?" I said.

He doesn't at all. He thinks it's hilarious. And he laughs. A wicked laugh. And he's right. It is funny.

"So when will the new stuff grow in?" he enquires. And I tell him in around four months.

"Do you know what? Speed it up at bit. Get one of those hydroponic lights and attach it to your head at night, that way it will make it grow faster."

I laugh. And then tell him I can't think about the new hair follicles growing yet. I'm still coming to terms with the transplanted hair shafts falling out.

"Put them under your pillow," he advises. "In the morning lift it up and you'll find a fringe."

I have to laugh. Again.

"Listen," he says, "think about how you'll feel when it all grows in. When you go out in your wee sports car you can let someone else drive."

"Eh? Why?"

"Because then you can spend all the time with your hair out the windae . . . all blowing in the wind for the world to see."

His voice becomes a little more serious.

"You're a brave man," he says. "You're the first person any of us know who's had the balls to have a hair transplant. I'm sure it will work out brilliantly."

Let's hope.

'A man can be short and dumpy
and getting bald but If he has
fire, women will like him.'

~ Mae West.

17
Caesar's Combover

I KNOW I should be trying to keep my head clear of hair thoughts, at least for some of the time, but it's hard. I can't pass a mirror without looking for signs of new growth. And even when I'm not thinking about hair popping up, the subject pops up. As it has right now, in my e-mail box.

It's an e-mail from the London 'tug n' plug' transplant company advertising their summer deals in Athens. The cost sounded reasonable, but I'm entirely glad I didn't go to Greece, Argentina or one of the Eastern European countries to have the HT carried out. I'd have felt I was flying blind into a foreign clinic. If it had all gone wrong I'd have felt the worst journalist in the world for not carrying out all the research, even if it's not easy researching clinics when they've been open much less time than a hair cycle.

As I'm reading the e-mail however I realise I'm touching my head. Not the donor area. I've forgotten all about that, although it's still a little itchy at times. But the top. Again. It's what I do. It's reassurance. It's hope. And I'm looking at my scalp in the mirror. Again.

It's the end of May and all of the transplanted hair has fallen off, gone like September leaves, and it will be months before it re-grows. But my original hair, which Dr Farjo shaved, has started to come back in. Little hairs. But hairs nonetheless. Everything is happening as it should. However, combined with the very short sides haircut, for now I look more bald than I did before the transplant. I look like Ivan Denisovich.

And that's why, as I'm walking down the street for a sandwich, I'm getting stares from people I haven't seen for a while. The sun is out and I'm tempted to get a little colour to the head. It looks so white. Yes, the bald look could be helped if the scalp were a little darker.

It reminds me of a chat with old pal, Bill. Balding in his twenties, before going out at night, (this was in the 1950s) he and his pals who were also thinning would touch the side of the chimney and coat their finger tips with soot. Then they'd touch up the bald spots.

Should I think about the modern-day equivalent, the cans of 'hair thickener' and 'scalp colouring' agents, the dry cosmetics which get rubbed into the scalp, made from chopped-up sheep hair which is grated into microscopic pieces, dyed and given a negative static charge so that it sticks to whatever hair remains?

These tins of spray-on hair that are hugely popular with TV presenters looking for a quick hair fix. But I don't fancy the idea of mocking up my own bare-ish scalp at the moment. What if you get caught in the rain? The chances of getting caught in the rain in Glasgow is greater than the chance of catching a verruca in a dirty swimming pool.

Okay, I'm bothered by the balding look - but I know it's temporary, that great new hair will appear.

It will. Won't it. For the moment I take comfort in knowing that mankind has been struggling with hair loss ever since he could see his own hair-lacking reflection in a pool of water.

The Hairfile reveals that ancient Egyptians treated baldness with a scalp treatment of equal parts of fat from a snake, a lion, a hippopotamus, a crocodile, a goose and an ibex. (Whatever an ibex is/was?) And in 1500BC the same nation developed a potion made up of the toes of a dog, dates, the hoof of an ass and the blood from the neck of a gagbu bird. (ditto.)

Not only would the ancient Egyptians have found no friends within animal welfare groups, they had to cope with the fact the treatments failed.

The Romans faired no better. And even their self-proclaimed gods were not immune to andro-genetic alopecia, or male pattern baldness as we call it these days. Roman coins show that Julius Caesar parted his hair just above one ear - and thencombed some pathetic long strands over the top of his head.

'I came, I saw, I combedover,' could have been his catch phrase.

Well, at least I never resorted to camouflage.

Caesar in fact tried all sorts of hair restoration treatments. His Queen of the Nile chum Cleopatra is said to have given the Roman god a ground-up compound of mice, horse teeth and deer marrow. (Again you really hope the horses were dead before they had their teeth extracted.)

And so the experimentation and false hope continued over the centuries. Hippocrates looked for a baldness cure. And he in fact stumbled onto something. He deduced that castration appeared to work. (Hopefully his experiments were volunteer-based.) Insecure men were desperate however to believe that baldness could be treated, which allowed for the differing versions of snake-oil salesman to appear (so-called because they did indeed bottle snake-oil at one time and pass it off as a treatment.)

And insecure women. Closer to home, Queen Victoria, who suffered from thinning hair, came up with her own antidote. She drank draughts of wine fermented from the sap of silver birch trees. Now it's unclear whether the libation actually helped her tresses to become thicker, although it's likely she at least smiled more often.

Yet, the search for the Holy Grail of hair restoration was unrelenting.

In 1908, John Breck, a chemist from Massachusettes, set out to cure his baldness by concocting a variety of hair potions. He became America's leading shampoo maker and died a millionaire in 1965.

But he was a bald millionaire.

And in 1995 researchers at Duke University, North Carolina, confirmed that castration *was* effective. But the researchers concluded that 'while castration may be a cure, it is not commercially viable.'

Who'd have thought it?

In recent years, manufactures however have attempted to sell us all sorts of products suggesting, not claiming (that would be illegal) that our hair health will greatly improved if used regularly. For a while it was product with amino acids included. Made sense. Sort of. After all aminos are the body's building blocks. Put them on your head and you've soon got an Empire State Building of hair?

Not really.

'Amino acids are meat,' said one leading dermatologist. 'If you think you can cure baldness with amino acids you might just as well walk around with a piece of meat slapped on your head.'

But, it turns out having a piece of meat stuck to your skull could help.

A little.

The placebo effect can work to a degree; you can never underestimate the mind's ability for self-delusion. And if the mind believes it, it can happen, to a tiny degree. If a bald man rubbed peanut butter or bull semen or mayonnaise on his head every night for three months, he might notice a few hairs responding.

'No one knows why this happens, but it does.'

But while chemists were continually experimenting with new product new hair transplantation techniques were being developed. And now, here we are in the middle of 2008, and transplants are now a success story the world over.

Last year, Americans alone - with New York City and Los Angeles leading the way - shelled out an incredible $1.2 billion for 100,445 hair restoration procedures. That's almost a 50% increase on procedures carried out in 2004.

And I can delight in those numbers. Most of these 100,445 must have had a good result - or bad press would have been the result. My transplant *will* give me new hair.

After considering the possibility for years, I can rest assured that I've made the right decision, I've chosen the very best possibility for my head.

Or have I?

18
The Shock Cure

IT'S six o'clock, June 2, and I'm driving home from work listening to the BBC's Five Live as usual - and suddenly I'm almost veering off the road. The lead story is a report of a new cure for baldness, citing hair cloning as the answer.

But it's not the content of the story that has me grasping at the wheel, it's the voice I'm listening to.

It's Dr Farjo.

Dr Bessam Farjo is on the radio talking about how this new technique will mean an end to baldness. What? Does that mean I've had 3,200 FUs implanted on my head for sweet FA?

The next day, the story, which had emerged from an international conference of hair replacement surgeons in Rome, is all over the papers.

David Rose in *The Times* reports; 'Millions of men and women who suffer from premature baldness or hair loss could soon be able to regain their original lustrous locks - by cloning their hair in the laboratory, research suggests.' Fantastic. It's great news for the balding.

'The new technique, known as "follicular cell implantation", has already shown positive results in continuing clinical trials on human beings.'

Great. But what about me?

'The latest results of the Phase II trial suggest that the technique can increase hair count in at least two thirds of patients after six months, and four out of five if the scalp is stimulated beforehand.'

Yes, yes, stimulate schwimulate. But have I jumped the gun? The story goes on to explain the process; cells are multiplied many times over in a special patented culture before being injected back into the scalp in their millions, stimulating the formation of new hair follicles or rejuvenating those that have stopped producing hair on the top of the head.

'It will be quicker and less invasive than current hair transplant techniques favoured by celebrities including Sir Elton John (sic) and Silvio Berlusconi, the Italian Prime Minster.'

And me. What about me?

'Bessam Farjo, who is leading the research, said that (very positive) results after six months were now available for 11 patients out of 19 currently enrolled on the trial.'

Wonderful. I'm delighted that it's Dr Farjo who is the top banana in the project. But I feel as thick as soft fruit at the moment. Why didn't Dr F tell me that a new, faster, shiny, more prolific option was on the way?

The Times story continued; 'About 3,000 transplants – costing between £2,500 and £7,000 – take place at private clinics in Britain every year.'

Yes. And I'm one of that number. I've had a hair transplant. And now hair transplants are practically redundant.

'Dr Farjo said that his team was also experimenting with combining the DP cells with keratinocytes - cells that produce keratin, the basic building material of hair - so that they could grow actual hairs for transplant, rather than injectable cells.

'This could further improve surgeons' control over the amount, direction and appearance of the transplanted hair.'

Wonderful. Stem cell-grown hair that's completely non-Don King.

But what about me? Well, as you can imagine, I'm on the phone to Mick faster than you can say dermal papilla.

"I was wondering if you'd heard Dr Farjo on the radio," he says with a smile in his voice.

"Yes, Mick. I did. And it's a fantastic new development."

"It will change the way hair is re-grown."

"Yes, and I'm presuming that the reason the world hasn't heard of Dr Farjo's new development (by 'the world' I mean me) is that it won't be available for some time?"

"That's exactly right. It's all at least five years away."

Phew. Well, I certainly didn't have another five years to wait.

But it is fantastic news. What, with transplants working now. (I hope). And stem cell treatments five to ten years along the road.

The men of the world need never fear being bald again. And I'm thinking that those who come up with the quack treatments and the shampoos and all the zany products must be having kittens.

Little fluffy, hairy, kittens.

'You can never remain a rock
n'roll star if you go bald. It just
wouldn't work.'

~ Oasis kingpin **Noel Gallagher**
when asked would brother Liam
survive as a frontman if he lost his
hair.

19
Jungle Hair

'IS she happy to be going out with such an extreme example of male vanity?'

That's not the actual question people ask, but it's what they mean when they say 'What does your partner think of you having it done?' (The other key questions they come up with are 'Will it definitely work?' 'How much did that set you back?' and 'Was it sore?')

The Blonde's position, as I've mentioned, has always been 'Go for it. I don't think you need it. But if you want it. . .'

Well, that's what she said. And if I were to put money on it I'd bet there's a part of her subconscious that wants to see me with (more) hair. There's a part that wants to see me younger looking. So perhaps she sees the fringe benefit to my new hairline. That's not to say however that problems will not emerge with your partner if you skip happily down the road to self-improvement.

A friend once told his partner he was going on a diet, he felt he needed to lose a few pounds because he was becoming more of a nine pack than a six- pack. But his girlfriend went in a huff. Why? She reckoned his weight control plan to cut down on the afternoon cakes at work was in effect holding a mirror up to her own Little Plum tum. She reckoned if he were so concerned with his own extra stomach space he must also be thinking about hers.

I know. Perverse. But we're Venus and Mars. Still, at least the Blonde seemed to have embraced the positives in my HT. Which set me thinking; perhaps if more women knew of the hair transplant process, there would be less unhappy bald men out there? After all, millions of men let there wives/partners buy their clothes for them, tell them what colours suit. Would – should – partners suggest their men should have new hair?

I'm thinking about this very notion when the office phone rings.

"That's five weeks since you've had your transplant," says Mick. (It's the first week in June.)

"Just wondered how it's all coming along?"

"Great, Mick. I've managed to get my head together, or at least Dr Farjo has. The stitches are all but gone you see. The tiny pieces of plastic compound have been coming away over the past few days, like little bits of artificial dandruff.

"But it's pleasant to know their presence is no longer required to hold my once-divided head in place."

"Great. Listen, I've just had a thought. Perhaps you would write a blog for the Hair Restoration Forum website? It's an independent website used by blokes who've had, or are thinking about having a transplant."

"Yes, I will Mick. "I've already been writing lots of thoughts down."

And as I speak a thought comes to me. Before I went through the transplant process I weighed up the pros and cons for about a year. It took me about that time to research, work up the courage and convince myself, family and friends I should go for it. Mmm.

"Mick, what if there were a book on the market that recorded and explained the process?

"I think it's a great idea!" he says, excitedly.

And now I'm excited by the idea. There's no doubt there is massive interest in the subject. You can't count the number of websites devoted to hair restoration/improvement/treatment. And the public – and the media – can't seem to get enough information about hair cover.

Once upon a time the focus was wigs. If a celebrity were discovered to be a wig wearing, this could make a tabloid splash, which is why Sinatra and Heston and Wayne went to great lengths never to be photographed uncoiffed. And it's why Uncle Chris used to cut Tony Bennett's remaining hair and work on his wig in secret locations in the dead of night.

This is also why Little Richard went undercover, figuratively and literally. (And of course Gary Glitter, though to be fair I interviewed him a couple of times and didn't see the join. Though, to be extra fair, there wasn't one. He used a full wig, not a piece.)

Now, the interest in wig wearing is still there. At the beginning of 2008 the *Daily Mail* ran pics of Sly Stallone 'wondering' if he'd had a weave. Rambo wearing a rug? Even a state-of-the-art, all singing-and-dancing impossible to remove rug? It certainly looks like it could be added hair.

Then I began to wonder more about Sly's hair state. Why not have a transplant? No, that wouldn't be enough for him. A Rambo needs to have jungle hair.

Yes, the media still want to know what's on a man's head. When actresses first began to have artificial breasts inserted, the newspapers would have a field day, revealing where the work had been done, and how much it cost.

Nowadays, it's hardly a story. In fact, a young less than well-endowed actress who refuses to have implants is more of a story. But Botox treatment and cosmetic surgery is still news because the public are making their own minds up whether to follow in the star's slipstream.

And so are celebrity hair transplants, because they're not that common. Or are they? And we just don't know it. But the point stands, men who are losing their hair don't know where to turn to for an independent commentary on the process. They need to have the hair transplant process demystified.

Mick is becoming more and more enthusiastic.

"A book would let guys out there know what it's really like," he says.

"And unlike some of the website commentators you can write. Plus, I can fill you in with any science detail you need."

"Fantastic," I say. "It's a wonderful opportunity to become even more self-obsessed than I am already."

20

Hats Cause Baldness

THE idea of writing continually about my hair adventure has a major plus. It somehow helps justify my Obsessive Compulsive Disorder.

A bit.

Which is exactly what I'm displaying right now watching the tennis. The Stellar Artois Tennis Tournament is on television, taking place in London. And it's not Andy Murray's chances I'm discussing with the Blonde.

Not that I don't care about the immensely talented young man whom I once beat at my own local club (okay, he was eight at the time), I do, but right now I'm more focused, or rather fixated, with Australian pop star/actor Jason Donovan. Jason isn't on court, but he's in the crowd. And he's a man who a few years back looked as though he were headed on a one-way ticket to Slaphead Central. Now, he looks to have a decent head of hair. A little sparse at the temples perhaps, but thick enough and very natural looking. Mmm.

Now, it would be unwise of me to suggest that the extremely litigious and very nice Mr Donovan has had some professional help with his hairline. But somehow he seems to have reversed his hair fortunes. And I say good on yer', mate.

The Blonde however says my hair-related OCD is getting worse. A short while ago when watching the Chelsea v Manchester United European Championships Final my eyes were drawn to Chelsea star Joe Cole. Not because of his magical soccer talent, but his hairline. Cole looks to have a serious balding spot on the back of his head.

So here's the point - yes, there is one - to my observations; I can understand why Prince Charles and his unfortunate heir William didn't take off to the transplant clinics as soon as the flash cameras begin to reflect off their heads - they don't want to be seen to have had work done, and they don't want to provide the press with juicy copy.

But Joe Cole? If you earn £120k a week, surely you don't need to have a bald spot large enough to accommodate the word Adidas? Why don't these guys, who earn squillions, do something about it? I'm struggling for an answer to that one because the likes of Aussie cricketer Graham Gooch publicises his hair weave. However, it seems that when it comes to hair transplantation most men (outside of North America) still live in the Dark Ages. They still consider that baldness is something you just have to contend with. And that's probably to do with the fact that only recently the media have come to consider men's personal improvement projects with any degree of positivity. Or have they? Have the media - people like me - always ridiculed the follicly challenged?

For the sake of research (and something to do to stop me thinking about my new hair growth) I decide to look back at how baldness has been reported over the years. And *The Times* of April 24, 1919 offers a fascinating insight into the bald 'facts' of a century ago. First up, baldness, back then, was put down to the flu.

The Medical Correspondent wrote; 'Attention has lately been caled (sic) to the fact that baldness among men is on the increase.

'The influenza epidemic has been blamed, and many other causes for example, the stress and strain of' war have been mooted.'

Then he (I presume it was a male writer) adds; 'This is the more remarkable when it is considered that baldness is really a very unsightly and distressing condition. There is assuredly a great, if not perhaps vital, need for scientific work upon it. It is as much and as legitimately an object of scientific work as any other of our common diseases.'

A man after my own heart.

'No one can afford to say that if this apparently simple malady were studied facts of value in other directions would not be forthcoming.'

Again, you're not wrong.

The Correspondent went on to note that when a man is 'completely bald' his hair as a rule remains quite thick for some distance above his ears and round the back of his neck. 'Yet the top of his scalp is then shiny and, in scientific language, atrophic.

'How to explain this?'

Well, doctors didn't know about DHT in those days. So what was the cause? Turns out it was the old favourite. Failure of blood supply to the top of the head.

And hats. Goodness. I've realised that men have making wild guesses about hair loss for ever. What's incredible to me however is that the men of the nation still wore hats for the four decades - even though this 'scientific' theory had appeared in the world's most prestigious organ.

Did no one read *The Times* at this time? What about the bowler hats who bought it every day? Was it too much of a fashion faux pas to ditch the hat – even if you thought it were causing the blood to stop flowing?

What's also fascinating is that it took the medical world a long time to move away from the 'hat' theory. But at least they have. Although they don't always seem to get baldness in perspective. An example is the recent writing of Stefan Pasternack, an associate clinical professor of psychiatry at Georgetown University's medical school.

'Some men focus on their baldness as a kind of screen onto which they can project most of their fears and self-doubts. One young man actually considered castration just to keep his hair.'

Scary. But believable. Then he adds however; 'For most men, baldness isn't a big deal, although you can get a sun-burn on your head, which is a bore. For others, baldness is a kind of displacement - a focus for their insecurities. You may say that a bald head is to a man what flabby arms are to a woman. The individual worries about it much more than society does.'

No. You're wrong on a couple of points there, Professor P. Women with flabby arms can take to the gym, lift some light weights while at the same time cutting down on the chocolate cake. There isn't a fitness centre in the world that will help balding men. And what do you mean 'much more than society does'. Men are part of society. And billions are bald and don't want to be. And of course 'society' loves to poke fun at those with shiny heads.

I tell the Blonde about my argument with the Prof's logic. She agrees bingo wings can never beat baldness. And it turns out she's becoming a little fixated with all things follicular too. No, that's not true. She's just humouring my obsession.

We're watching television and John Travolta appears on a TV news clip. Gosh, I swear he had less hair the last time I saw him on TV, which was only a few weeks ago. Can't have been a transplant. The result looks all too much like that achieved by Robin Gibb of the Bee Gees.

But if Travolta did have some work done you can understand why. He can't become bald. He needs hair. He wouldn't have landed the *Saturday Night Fever* role had he been thin on top. He wouldn't have become a *Reservoir Dog* had he not had the requisite amount of fur on his head. He needed hair to push back, to grease, to play with.

Remember, only the very bad guys, who invariably get killed in the end, are bald. And by way of confirmation I've just picked up on a report about the new *Star Trek* movie. According to Trek Movie.com the Romulan villains will all be bald. Actor Eric Bana is having his head shaved for his part as one of the bad guys.

"There. Proof positive," I'm telling the Blonde, even though she's not even pretending to be interested.

"Don't believe me? Then show me a movie where the entire male content of a malevolent planetary force have a nice thick demi-wave, a clever gelled style, a Tony Curtis (Forties T.C.) or a neat line in frosted tips."

I pause for reflection and add; "Wonder if I'll every have enough hair for some frosted tips?"

"Wonder if you've really lost the nut," she says.

'Pete, did you know that men with hair earn 70 per cent more than their bald counterparts?.'

~ Hit sitcom *30 Rock's* insensitive and particularly demanding character Donaghy, played by **Alec Baldwin**, telling his bald employee why he should have new hair.

21
Yonda Lies My Hairpiece

OKAY, I've made the right move in having a hair transplant. But when will I see the results? It's now seven and a half weeks in and I'm showing concern. Why? No real reason. No unreal reason either. It's just that I've had so many people say to me 'What if it doesn't grow in?' that I'm starting to question the process.

It's got me thinking that perhaps I'm expecting too much. This worrying thought sticks with me like a summer cold and so the next day I call Mick. As always, he says the right thing.

"Be patient. It will appear."

No doubt he's been through this process of reassurance a thousand times, but you can't tell from his upbeat voice. He's always encouraging. In another life he would make an excellent counsellor.

Sadly, the thoughts of poor hair aren't allowed to exit my head. Tonight I'm watching a TV show I SkyPlused a couple of months back, *The Graham Norton Show*. I'd recorded it because Hollywood Tony Curtis was the star guest.

Now I'm thinking the star should have been counselled

on what to wear. On his head. Curtis has been wearing a wig longer than an aged barrister and now he's decided to come clean, whip it off and show the world his Daddy Warbucks.

It doesn't look good, Tony. In fact, it's frightening, allied to what looks like a face-lift. It's a terrifying wake-up call to the ravages of time/Hollywood excess. We all want to remember you as you were, snogging Marilyn in *Some Like It Hot*, or fighting Kirk Douglas in *The Vikings* and muttering, in perfect Bronx-Scandinavian the immortal line 'Yonda lies da castle of my fadda'.

I know you are 83 and you have the perfect right to declare your comfortability with the fact you have nothing on top. But you can't be that comfortable, or you'd have bared all years ago.

In my condition however Curtis is making me uncomfortable. Why? I suppose if I'm honest I'm hoping I don't end up like Tony. I'm desperately hoping this transplant works out and I don't have to resort to other options, only to abandon them when I'm so old I think it doesn't matter.

And I'm confused. This is a man who was once one of the busiest men in Tinseltown, who has loved thousands of women and yet he's never had the balls to try a hair transplant?

And I'm getting slightly anxious. Well, not anxious, exactly. More a little confused. The original hair on my scalp is growing back in, but there seems to be more of it than before. Is this just my imagination? Is it wishful thinking? Is it just that I had absolutely nothing six weeks ago and comparatively, it looks far better?

A bit of research reveals that scalp hair grows about half

an inch a month (women's hair grows faster than men's) and the hair on the top of the head grows a little faster than the hair on the sides. So that accounts for the length. And it all grows faster in summer than in winter. (Perhaps there is a case for using the hydroponic light attachment on the head after all.)

But what about the thickness? It seems a fair bit thicker. Yet Mick says it can't be. The new hair can't have grown in yet. And it can't be down to the Finasteride. That can take a year to kick in.

Is the old hair thicker because it has been shaved? No. Most website advice centres say if you shave off the desperately thinning hair and hope for it to grow back in you've more of a chance of seeing Sinatra make a comeback.

Oh well. What I do uncover in this hair research is some fairly useless but fascinating information. (For someone with Hair OCD like me.) For example, a plug of hair removed from the scalp can live for three weeks without you if its roots are kept in a saline solution.

Now, my first thought on reading this is that one day the thick-haired men of the world will able to bequeath their hair to someone else, like a set of Steinbeck books. Sadly, however, not at the moment. Our body would take one look at the foreign hair cells and reject them, like a six year old being offered up semolina.

But then another fact makes me smile. I discover that hair grows for about 48 hours after you die. And that cracks me up. We are all worrying about losing our hair during our lifetime and yet when we shuffle off it still sprouts, in sheer bloody defiance.

How twisted is that?

But I really had to laugh when I read about the American company who opened a 'Hairbank' in 2002. Most of the major TV stations such as such as CNN and CBS News carried the story about this new technique in which men re-grow their own hair. It was based on the assumption that one day scientists will cure baldness by simply extracting DNA samples from our own hair. Nothing wrong with that. But in the interim, Hairogenics offered to provide a 'service' to the balding by offering to preserve a hair sample in a controlled environment, in Portland Oregon, until such time that the hair can be regrown.

No, read on. It gets better.

The company would take hair samples, vacuum-seal them in waterproof packages and then bury them underground. (Hairogenics cited that the Oregon soil had been proven by archaeologists "as the best, natural preservative for human DNA material.")

Brilliant. Someone will stick your hair in a poly bag and put it in a hole in the dirt, and all for just $59.95.

Not surprisingly, a barrage of the news station's website readers such as John saw the flaws in the hair-raising theory that the broadcasters didn't seem to spot.

'A strand of hair is made up only of dead cells and keratin. It's the cells in the follicle that matter.'

What was fascinating about the story however was the willingness of the TV stations to cover it. Stories about hair loss solutions are bankers, absolute guarantees in every form of the media because editors know there are bald men waiting to hear of the discovery of the Holy Grail of Hair.

Men like me. Yet, right now what I want to know is what's going on on my head.

'He's the kind of guy that when
he dies he's going up to heaven to
give God a bad time for making
him bald.'

~ **Marlon Brando,** on
Frank Sinatra.

22
Fretful Tufts

IT'S almost the end of July, almost three months since my HT, and I'm still touching my head more often than a priest during mass. But it's not that I'm worried. Sitting here at my office desk I can feel lots of spiky little hairs. It's not new hair of course. Mick says it can't be. It's too soon. No, it's some of the old hair making a comeback. And it's fantastic because each little spiky hair represents hope. And reassurance. And I need it, especially when I look at the hairs in the shower tray in the morning.

At least I can tell myself that it's just old hair that's been pushed out of the pram to make way for the new babies that will be born any minute. They will, won't they Sarah? Sarah is 27 and has a low boredom threshold.

Or perhaps it just seems she has.

She's now bored of taking pics of my head on her mobile phone. In fact, she's bored of any mention of my head.

"Do you see any new growth yet, Sarah?"

"No."

"Could those little spikys be new hair?"

"No."

"Look, I know you see my head every single day. So maybe perhaps you don't realise it's growing."

"It's still the same."

"Perhaps you're too scalp-familiar."

"No. It's still not grown."

"I brought you toast this morning, Sarah. And you still don't see signs of new hair?"

"No."

"And I gave you half a banana."

At this point I show her pics of me before the HT. (Yes, more OCD behaviour.)

"No, you don't look like you've got any more hair," she says.

And my face suggests I'm a little miffed. It wouldn't have hurt her to lie. A little. However, she picks up on this and offers her own form of encouragement.

"Have a look at this website," she says directing me to a site called Cressheads.

"It's for parents who need to find things to do for their kids. The idea is you put watercress seeds into an eggshell and then water it and it grows. Then you draw a little face on the eggshell when the cress hair has grown in.

"Just think of your new hair as watercress!"

Thanks, Sarah. But the cress seeds germinate in a couple of days. I've got to wait another month. At least. And sprinkling my head with water and putting it out on a window sill isn't going to speed up the process one little bit. Believe me, if I thought it did I would.

That's not to say I can't deal with having no hair. I can, for the present, in the sound knowledge the new hair will arrive. But being born with a defective patience gene, I'm finding it hard to sit and wait for Dr Farjo's work to take effect. 'How poor are those that have no patience! What wound did ever heal but by degrees,' wrote Shakespeare.

Well, it's not the wound that's bothering me, Willie. That's all healed up nicely. There is no numbness on the scalp at all. And you couldn't find the scar on the back of my head with a lens the size of a supermodel's bedroom mirror.

No, it's the waiting. And the wondering. I'm starting to think hard about what sort of result I can expect. I know the transplanted hairs looked great on HT Day, but what if they don't all come back?

I know others have had great results but some I've seen have looked all too ordinary. I'm all too aware that heads are like fingerprints; everyone is different. We've all got very different donor areas with varying densities. What sort of final covering will my transplant produce?

I don't want my Elmer Fudd head for too much longer. I want a decent head of hair. I was at a 50th birthday party on Saturday and again the chat from those with hair was about exactly that.

And I need comfort. It's back to the Hairfile. Which reinforces the notion that men have been awful to each other about hair loss ever since they developed the language to convey it.

Take last century for example. You would have thought that Britain's menfolk were too busy worrying about World Wars, rickets, pneumonia and Vera Lynn-induced ear ache to criticise those with less hair. Not true according to *The Times*, of April 3, 1939. Our readiness to mock the hairless abounded even then.

The paper's Medical Correspondent wrote a column based on the news that 'a gentlemen' left a large sum of money in his will; £400, to two hospitals, to be used to find out the causes and remedies of 'seasickness, post-nasal catarrh - and, (get this) baldness.'

The colourful writer then speculates as to the merits of the nice old fellow's bequest. And his comments are revealing.

'It is easy to feel sorry for the seasick; and it is particularly easy to feel sorry for them if you are yourself immune to their qualms. Limp, green, and groping, they provide just the contrast you need as you stride with discreet insouciance upon the heaving deck. You feel for them, at the least, the ignoble pity that goes with condescension.

'It is the same with catarrh, whether post-nasal or not. Sneezes are music to the germ-proof man, and here again a certain sympathy goes out to the streaming noses and the fuddled consonants of those lesser creatures whose plight throws into his own vulnerability.'

Then he continues, with the all-important line; 'But the bald? Are the hirsute automatically sorry for the bald? They feel, no doubt, SUPERIOR to them, but it had not, until now, appeared that this superiority implied compassion.'

And what he adds, this Times Medical Corr of 1939, is that they don't deserve it either. (It's just as well you're long dead, mate.)

'The process by which a man loses his hair is - if it is natural – is painless.'

Then he seems to be having a laugh.

'Bald men, after all, pay no barber's bills. They need buy no unguents with which to master their hair, no shampoos to conserve its lustre, no silver-backed brushes to clutter up their dressing-tables.'

He continues; 'Their suitcases are lighter than those of hairy men, and their hearts ought to be lighter too, for their responsibilities are fewer. The pleasing refulgence of their polished skulls ought really to be token contentment in at least one department of their life. Lucky fellows!'

Lucky? How so?

'Never again to endure, swaddled and helpless, the political opinions of a barber; never again with nervous hands to smooth, on the threshold of a strange drawing-room, that fretful tuft which a hasty toilet overlooked.'

Endure opinions? I'll have you know I quite enjoyed my chats with Sheenya about her finding herself on the first night of a holiday and on a foreign beach and skinny dipping and someone stealing all her clothes and having to make her way back to the hotel bare-naked - but not remembering where her hotel was because the address was in her stolen handbag. I quite liked sorting my hair out in any drawing-room, strange or not.

But what I take from reading this piece is not just an insight into the journalism of the day or that the bloke was a very clever writer with a lovely turn of phrase, it's an absolute confirmation that men have always either felt sorry for those with less hair - or taken the mickey at every opportunity.

Or both. It's affirmation that those with hair aren't happy enough just to have it. They need to make fun of those who don't. But now, at least I can take comfort from the fact that men like me can have their silver-backed brushes cluttering up every inch of their dressing-tables should they feel like it.

They can. Can't they?

23
Brian Boru

I NEVER thought I'd every hear myself mutter the phrase 'God I wish I were dense.' But I am. I want more hair. Thicker hair.

A couple of days have gone by since reading the *Times* man's comments, which seemed to somehow make me even more focused on my head. I need distraction. I've tried the summer movies but they don't work. *Sex and the City* had a paint-by-numbers script and Steve Carell was massive disappointment in *Get Smart*. In fact, if Mel Brooks, who wrote the original TV series were dead, he'd be spinning in his grave right now.

So what to do? I just want to see the result of this hair work so much I'm wishing the days away. And at the risk of sounding all melodramatic, there's a hair movie currently playing in my head. Or more specifically it's playing one scene where calendar pages are blown off by a powerful wind; you know the old device used by film directors in the Forties to indicate the rapid passage of time.

But this Capra-esque scene is slightly different because each calendar page has a photo of me with a bald head imprinted on it. And when the last page falls to the ground like a feather, the camera than pans across to show an aerial view of my head, which has a lovely covering of hair. All that's missing from the scene is a log fire, a thick cardigan and a big yellow Labrador sitting at my feet.

Yes, I'm going soft in the head. I've even thought of a song or a poem title which highlights my state of mind. *All I Want For Christmas Is A Comb*. I confess this to my talented writer chum Ian and a couple of hours later he sends me an email with a poem attached. (See Last Page.) It really makes me smile. And it makes me think positively of my new Christmas hair. I've even decided upon the comb I'll buy. The Rolls Royce of combs. A new tortoiseshell Stratton hair comb.

Yes, that's the focus of my thoughts now. Let's just hope it has something to comb. But what to do meantime? I need to share my head thoughts with the empathetic. If you go into hospital to have a piece of cartilage debris removed from your knee, mention it in the tennis club changing room a couple of weeks later and there will be five guys who've undergone the same procedure. Yet, mention you've had a hair transplant to the unknowns - not that I have - and I do know it would either attract wry grins or stares of disbelief.

Thankfully, Mick comes up with the answer. He suggests I post my 1,000 word blog onto the *Hair Restoration Forum* (hairtransplantnetwork.com) a website for those who've had a transplant, or are thinking about having one.

And it sounds a great idea. After all, here is a chance to connect with others who've gone through the whole worrying – or hopefully invigorating–process.

And visiting the *Forum* is a fascinating experience. Suddenly, my comment on the procedure is being read by blokes in Omaha, Orlando and London. Here on the *Forum*, everyone is of a common purpose - the pursuit of new hair.

Most are agreed transplant is the answer; it's a question of how, when, where, how much - and what kind of result can you expect.

Yet, what's important about the website is the sense of community it creates. Men, in general, are not great when it comes to sharing anxieties, especially something so vanity-based as a baldness fear. And this *Forum* offers an outlet.

Okay, those who join the *Forum* get to remain anonymous, and can choose electronic pen names such as *Spex and Badger*. (Mine is *Brian Boru*, not because I see myself as the legendary King of Ireland, but because a fellow hospital patient once did a drawing of me when I was a wee boy, which I still have, and entitled it *Brian Boru*).

However, it's interesting to read the bold, direct comments coming in, which vary from being informed to erudite to simplistic.

Balody, who also been given new hair by Dr Farjo, read my tale and declared; *Wow! That was an epic review! It mirrored my Farjo experience to the T , even the same sandwich.*

Falc was equally postive; *Congratulations on selecting a first-rate surgeon. We could almost make a movie out of your experience. But in the midst of all that detail, I didn't catch how many grafts you received. I also hope that you'll share your photos and document your progress with us by creating a hair loss weblog.*

Ooops. They want details. And photos. Of course they do. These guys offer up the tiny detail of their own experience and expect the same. Some even offer personal information, about where they live, their baldness experience etc.

Dewayne went on to reveal the number of hair plugs (50) he'd had removed after a transplant in 1991, which were replaced by 2750 FU's in 2008.

He even listed his current regimen for hair recovery; *1.25 mg Proscar M-W-F, (Monday, Wednesday and Friday) Rogaine 5% Foam - once daily, AndroGel, once daily, Lipitor 5 mg every other day.*

Wow. That's an awful lot of effort to add hair to your head. And I realised that the people on this site are every bit as focused on hair recovery as I am. No, that's not true at all. My interest in re-growing hair is almost incidental by comparison. These guys are hardcore hair transplantees.

And it's really a delight to know that that there are millions of others out there who are even more mentally deranged than me. But would I have used the site alone as a basis for making a judgement about which surgeon I chose? I don't think so. It's certainly an indicator; you'd be crazy to ignore half a dozen negative comments about a particular doctor. And on the other hand, it would be pointless to ignore a list of herograms for a nominated surgeon.

Yet, it's hard to glean a definitive judgement from a bloke who's reduced to a single name in italics. And given that it's an international website, much of the input is American (because most transplants are carried out in the States). And criteria can vary, I reckon. We're all in the pursuit of more hair, but does someone who's just had a HT in Indian Wells or Indianapolis have the same expectation as me? Are we coming from the same cost base?

Still, at least I've found a comfort zone, a place where I can go share in the experience. And it's helped me focus. I'm calm. Especially when I discover one posting from *Spex,* bless him, who told me exactly what I needed to hear.

Patience is the toughest part of the HT procedure but one of the most important ones; looking constantly in the mirror, inspecting it (at) every opportunity, driving along staring in the rear view mirror (how I never crashed I don't know).

Wondering why at exactly 3/4 months there is still no growth! Be prepared post op to really make a conscious effort to put it all on the back burner for 6 months as a bench mark as other wise you will only drive yourself MAD! - Trust me - I speak from personal experience!!'

Well, at least I don't have redness. Never did. Although I have looked in the rear view mirror myself a few too many times. And in shop window reflections. In fact, anywhere there is glass. In fact, I don't even need glass. A dirty puddle will do.

However, thanks to the visit to the *Forum* I'm relaxed now.

I can wait for my new hair.

Well, I think I can.

'The rheumatic singer who de-
fied doctors and male-pattern
baldness to become a star.'

~The Internet Movie Data Base
summary of **Bobby Darin** who,
incidentally, wore a hairpiece.

24
Curb Your Angst

IT'S now three months post HT and I'm starting to panic. Forget about what the blokes on the *Hair Restoration Forum* said about being patient. It said on the Farjo post-op leaflet that the new hair would start to grow in three/four months time. Well, it's now 12 weeks. In fact, it's 84 days and six hours to be exact since the last follicle was inserted into my head. And what have I got to show for it? Not a lot. I think.

My two sisters tell me every week that they can see new life appear and of course they are now experts. Every Sunday they pull my mother's Woolworth's magnifying glass out of the drawer to get a good look at my head and they say they can see lots of little hairs appear.

"It's definitely growing. And it looks thicker," says Maureen, comfortingly.

"Are you sure?"

"Well, it's certainly longer. And there's more of it."

"No, you're imagining it."

"No, she's not," says Anne. "You've got more hair than you had before the transplant. In fact, if you didn't grow any more hair at all you could be pleased with the amount that's there now."

"No, you're being daft. It can't have grown in. Can it?"

I don't think they are being daft. I *want* to think it's thicker. But I'm not entirely sure so I'm playing Devil's Advocate to a degree. Now, you'd think I'd know whether or not I have more hair on my head than my March hair state. But I'm genuinely not sure. It looks more, but I spoke to Mick recently about this and he said the new hair can't have grown in already – not to any degree worth noticing, anyway.

"It's too soon," he says of the new forest.

"You'll be looking at five months before you start to see a result. And then it could keep on growing up to a year because the different hair follicles grow at different rates."

So am I delusional? Are my sister's caught up in a demi-wave of optimism? Mmm. But there's another fact to consider. I reckon I waited until the very last minute before having the transplant. In fact, I waited about six months beyond the very last minute. As a result I had very little left up top. And what I did have was disappearing faster than Hilary Clinton's nomination chances.

And in the days before transplant I reckoned that what was left would only survive another few months, four or five at most. This simple arithmetic meant that without the transplant it all adds up to the fact I'd be headed right into Shineyhead territory by now. But I'm not. According to the Joyful Sisters the hairline is getting thicker.

Confused? You bet I am.

So here's a chance for an independent overview. It's now August 1st and I'm having my fourth Vinnie haircut. (I guess Sheenya is too caught up with Mary-Kate and

Ashley during the school holidays to wonder about my new hair.) Vinnie however is delighted with the result so far.

"It really looks thicker," he says, lifting up hair at the back with his comb as he searches for the scar line, which he is finding very hard to locate.

"Yes, Vinnie, but it's not due to start growing until around now. This is probably just the original hair growing back in.

"Who cares?" says Vinnie. "It looks good. Ah. Found the scar. Gosh, you can hardly see it at all."

I try to look at it, with the benefit of two cleverly angled mirrors. Yes, I can see the scar. But it's more faint than an actress at an awards ceremony.

Now, I'm looking onto the top of my head. Are those new hairs or just old ones making one emboldened, final re-appearance, like an aged movie star? It's hard to tell. I want to believe Vinnie but . . .

The Blonde, meantime, is sick of me asking her about the state of my skull.

"It's exactly the same as it was the last time you asked me," she says, throwing a javelin of disinterest right at me.

And I make a point to take that disinterest and toss it right back at her at some point - the next time she asks what I think of her new hair-do, for example.

"And will you stop touching your head," she adds. "It won't make it grow any faster."

"Yeh? How do you know? How do you know that there isn't an energy involved in touch and in some way I am encouraging growth?"

She looks at me as though I'm daft. And perhaps I am.

So I try to prove her wrong. I go away and read up on theories which suggest that an energy exchange of some type occurs between individuals. And I find one.

Apparently, touch energy is a central theme in many healing techniques. The heart, for example, generates a strong electro-magnetic field and when people touch electro-magnetic energy is exchanged. Electro Cardiograph machines can actually measure it. So who's to say when I touch my head I'm not transferring energy, ergo stimulation to my follicles? And who's to say that ESP doesn't exist, that by touching and thinking about hair growth on my head I'm not willing it to grow?

I present this new, reasoned, inarguable evidence to her. And she takes a moment and delivers her considered, reasoned, reply.

"You're bonkers," she says.

And just to underline the point adds; "Get a life."

Perhaps she's right. Luckily for me I have the collapse of the world banking systems, the rocketing cost of energy, global warming and terrorism to dwell upon or I would be completely OCD about the hair not coming in. And I put it all in perspective. The new hair will arrive. It will. It will. And I'm telling myself this as I'm making breakfast, waiting for the kettle to boil, which is next to the cooker. What's that smell? It's the toast! But as I turn my head and race in the direction of the toaster, to my right, my head stops moving. It's because it's come up against an immovable object in the form of the sharp-sided cooker hood.

And the top of my head, about an inch from the front of my scalp, has lost the contact battle. It's painful. So painful in fact I would probably cry if I thought there were anyone around to give me attention. But the pain is not my main concern. When you've just had a hair transplant you immediately think about collateral damage.

This isn't about a bash to the brain. I've had lots of those before, being hit with footballs, football boots etc. No, this is about potential damage to the hair follicles in that area. Have I caused a few to fall out? Will they die off as a result of the sudden impact?

Gingerly, I'm touching the spot that took the direct hit. It's bad. I can feel a wetness. Yes, it's blood. Damn. It's getting worse. More blood. It's not trickling down, but there's enough so's I have to dab my head a few times before tackling my porridge. But now as I'm dabbing I'm laughing. If anything, the seeping blood proves that the baldness/lack of blood supply to the head theory is improbable. My head is clearly not short of blood, as this little red Niagara now proves.

Yet, I'm concerned about this damage. Have I lost a few FUs? I finish breakfast and hit the *Hair Restoration Forum*. I need to be told to relax and be patient. And there listed in the *True Experiences* section is the comfort I need.

Several bloggers point out that the hair follicles are so deeply imbedded by this point it would take a scalpel to remove them. The sharp end of a cooker hood doesn't have the same incisive capability. But going onto the *Forum* makes me think about Mick.

Yes, my *Before* and *After* pics. Mick has the *Befores*. Should I get him to send them? Should I get new pics taken so's I can compare? No, not yet. I'm not sure there will be much of a change. And although Mick's a sympathetic bloke I can't expect him to lie to me to make me feel better. In any case, if I tell him I need an urgent comparison he'll laugh his own head off. That's what I need to do. Laugh. To take my mind off my head.

Thankfully, Ian has lent me his *Curb Your Enthusiasm* box set and I love it, in the way you love to watch the ice skating reality shows when the diva-like soap actress falls flat on her giant axel.

The lead character in *CYE*, Larry (Larry David), is both excruciating and funny. One ep is titled *The Grand Opening*. But there's a surprise in store about five minutes in. Larry spots Phil, the bald chef he's hired in the restaurant. But Phil is wearing a toupee. And Larry feels compelled to fire him. Larry, you see, is bald. Very bald. But claims to be proud of his lack of hair. But this can't be true of course or he wouldn't have given a fig if Phil had chosen to wear a guardsman's helmet on his head. Larry however explains to his distraught restaurant partners that the chef had to go because he was literally a bald-faced liar.

Larry, incidentally, gets his come-uppance because the replacement chef he chooses, who has hair, also has Tourette's. Now, I'm laughing at the comedy set up which suggests the theory that (some) bald men need the reassurance that they are not alone - even if like Larry they wish they still had it. But I'm also laughing at the fact I've picked a comedy DVD to forget about hair issues - and came up with one in which the central theme is the psychology of baldness.

Still, at least I'm not going to become a Phil. I've got hair.

It's just that I'm not sure if you can see it at the moment.

25

Foghorn Leghorn Hair

"STOP touching yourself!" yells Sarah.

We're in the office of course, it's now August 13th, three and a half months after the HT and everyone turns round to see whom she's referring to. It's me of course. My colleague's command is by way of letting me know that I'm fingering my scalp once too often. Well, perhaps more than once.

It's only 11am and she informs she's counting how many times I touch my head and noting it down. Every fourth stroke she puts a line through the middle, like she were counting sheep through a pen. She reveals the paper with the lines on it. I count eleven.

Now Sarah, and the Blonde of course, reckon the OCD is progressing from minor to mid-range.

"I know you think your head is the magic lamp and if you rub it you will get your wish for more hair," says Sarah. "But you won't.

"You'll just get spots."

Caught. Bang to rights. I need a plan. What if I try to forget about the hair for a week? That would mean not seeing my head for a whole seven days. And there is an advantage to that idea. It would mean I'd have a clearer idea after the week if the hair had grown. But is it possible not to see your scalp for that length of time?

My imagination runs with the difficulties. There's morning shaving/tooth brushing for a start. I suppose I could wear a baseball cap. And I don't have to look in the mirror to dry my hair. It's not that I've got to style it or anything. Yet.

But what about the huge mirror in the dressing room at the tennis club? Or the one in the company toilet. Should I take to wearing a bandana? No, get over yourself. And it could be a bit difficult writing a book about the hair transplant process while not looking in the mirror.

Later that night I throw the mini dilemma at Ian over a pizza.

"Don't worry about the worrying," he says. "Just go with the flow. So what if you've become a self-obsessed lunatic? At least you have a sense of purpose in life."

His words of comfort didn't stop there.

"You're looking younger," he says.

Younger? The word sticks in my head.

"How do you mean."

"Well, the added hair makes you look younger."

The amazing thing is I feel he's being honest, and not just trying to make me feel better. Younger. What an incredible word! What a concept to embrace. When you go for new hair part of the reason is because having less hair ages you. You look older than your years. But axiomatically, and I never really thought about this, the opposite must be true. More hair on a man's head - than he has had in recent times - could make him look younger.

With a transplant I'd hoped to look just about right for

my age, but when you think about it most men of my age are either bald or quite thinning. If I'm neither I'll look younger. Wow!

Those with HTs certainly do look younger according to Dr. Paul Cotterill, president of the International Society of Hair Restoration Surgery of Geneva, Illinois.

'On average, you look eight to 10 years younger,' said the doc, of those who get new hair.

Well, if he's right, and I do have added hair on my head, not just the old stuff making a return visit, I *could* look younger.

Meantime, Ian and me throw around this notion, that I'm turning into Dorian Grey, Narcissus, Ursula Andress in *She*. And then we laugh when we think about it that none of these examples are so great. They're all parables for self-obsession. In *She* the lovely Ursula ended up a wizened old crone.

Still, let's push that aside for the moment. Adding hair is not just about protecting your head from the ravages of future time, it's about taking your appearance back a few years. What a fantastic notion. I'd long assumed that only two things improve with age; wine and Lulu. But now, my head can be included.

Just think about it. A few months ago I was becoming seriously irritated by wind. Not the gastro-entrological expulsion of air we all suffer from, now and again. No, *the* wind. And when it blew I'd feel the few wisps of hair that I had lift up and stay up. I looked like a balding rooster. And I was so aware of this Foghorn Leghorn look that I'd take the lift up to the office because it contained a mirror. And that offered me about 30 seconds to pat my few hairs into place. Now, if what Ian is saying is true, I won't have to head pat ever again. Now, for the next six months, or perhaps even longer, I can look forward to looking in the mirror in the morning.

And if all looks well enough, and the hair thickens, I won't have to touch my head fifty times a day for reassurance. Sarah won't have to record my OCD.

Ian, however, makes a point which could explain the scalp fingering.

"It may not be about what it's about," he says.

"Go on . . ."

"Well, you've had a major disappointment this year. Your expected showbiz legend biography was a major anticipation in your life (which I'd taken six years to write, only for the actor to change his mind at the last minute about publication) but when it was cancelled your spirits dropped dramatically.

"Shortly afterwards, you had the hair transplant. Perhaps this head involvement is displacement activity?"

I think for a while and reckon he's not wrong.

"But at least the registering of disappoint only manifests itself in touching my head and staring in glass – and talking about the new hair incessantly, I suppose."

"Yes, and you're also writing it all down. You're sharing the experience. You're letting other blokes know what they can expect from a hair transplant.

"It's all cathartic. It's a win-win."

26
Metrosexualised

I LEAVE the restaurant feeling quite pleased with my-self, quite cocky. And the next morning I take this cock-yness off to the dentist. Alastair looks at my head - hard not to when looking down at me in the chair.

"Yes, it's coming on," he says of the transplant, making me feel more upbeat.

"You don't look quite so ugly as you did last time."

"Great, Alistair. Now all you have to do is sort out my teeth."

"Why? They're fine."

"Yes, they are. Except one. And it's the front tooth. Or rather the new cap on the front tooth."

"What's wrong with it?"

"It's too big. What's the point of an expensive hair transplant that makes me look years younger and shock-ingly more handsome only to have the effect negated by a cap that's too lumpy?"

"It's not too lumpy at all."

"Don't get me wrong. It's a fine tooth. But it looks as though it should belong in someone else's mouth. It's a Bruce Banner of a tooth, after he turns green and Hulks up a bit of course."

"Okay, we'll make you a new crown."

And he does. And it's a fine crown. But the process makes me wonder if the progression towards looking younger is seeing me demand more from my dentist? I've had bulbous(ish) crowns (two) before and not batted an eyelid.

Has my personal vanity gland become over-active? And if it has, am I bothered?

The Sunday Times this week has an interesting feature that touches on that very subject. It's based on extracts from Kathleen Parker's book, *Saving The Male*. The author argues that women have been pressuring men for so long to become preened and perfect that they are in real danger of losing their maleness. Parker writes; 'In the process of fashioning a more female-friendly world we have created a culture that is hostile towards males, contemptuous of masculinity and cynical about the delightful differences that make men irresistible, especially when something goes bump in the night.'

Gosh? Does that mean my vanity project is about trying to fit in to this female-friendly world? It's women after all who traditionally have cosmetic surgery, treatments to improve their looks. Am I going all metrosexual to fit in with the image I think women want to see, when the reality is they're quite happy to see blokes unshaven, bald and wearing a *Die Hard* dirty vest?

Parker adds: 'The exemplar of the modern male is the hairless (on his body, not his head) metrosexualised man and decorator boys who turn heterosexual slobs into perfumed ponies. All of which is fine as long as we can dwell happily in the kingdom of Starbucks, munching our biscotti and debating whether nature or nurture determines gender identity. But in the dangerous world in which we really live it might be nice to have a few guys around who aren't trying to juggle pedicures and highlights.'

Well, I'm not that keen on biscotti, or Starbucks as it happens. The de-caff cappuccino always seems a little too tart for my taste. But has the excess oestrogen in the atmosphere affected my thinking?

Okay, I know I'm not a typical Alpha Male, I am a bit bookish and I do glance at the *Style* magazines at the weekend and use an Aloe Vera-based deodorant. But at the same time I loved rope swings as a kid, especially when they hung out over deep, dangerous swollen rivers, I've broken countless bones playing sports and skied down mountains without knowing how to stop.

Yes, I sound like I'm protesting too much. But honestly, having a HT is not about me trying to look better for women. If anything, it's more to do with looking better for men. Even Gordon. The next day in the office my reporter colleague hears Sarah mentioning my head count for the day, walks over, looks down at my head and says "Yes, your hair is getting longer."

Longer? Longer? So what? What kind of compliment is that? Well, it's not a compliment. It's damning with very faint praise. And my antennae is up to such comment now. You see, Gordon is around the same age. And he has quite thick hair. And blokes with thick hair who aren't very close friends don't *really* want to see others grow new hair. A transplant brings about a state of hair equality.

Gore Vidal's famous quote 'It's not enough that I succeed. Others need to fail.' is entirely apposite. In any case, I don't want long hair. Well, I do. But I want thicker hair that I can grow longer if I choose.

"Your hair's long but it's a bit fine," adds Gordon, sensing my upset but nevertheless continuing to dig an even deeper hole. Fine. Thanks a bunch. Which makes me think where did the expression 'fine hair' come from? There's nothing fine about 'fine' hair. It's hair that's thin.

And that's it. Look, I know that shampoo makers aren't going to bottle their gunk with labels saying *Especially for thin, pathetic, soon-to-be-gone Foghorn Leghorn rooster hair*. But a little honesty would be good.

Thankfully, I can always count on Robert for that. My theatre producer pal is as direct as 'Next!'

"The hair is really coming on," he says, over lunch, his comment unsolicited.

"Thanks."

"You know, you look so much younger already."

"Eh?"

"Yes, you look younger. You don't look your age. Now."

"Well, thanks. But aren't you the little bastard who six months ago said to me I didn't need a hair transplant? 'Just get it all cut short,' you said. 'It's all the fashion anyway'."

"Yes, I did. But what I was really trying to say was that you're pathetic attempts to keep it long and hide your white scalp all seemed a bit tragic.

"I reckoned you'd be better doing the honest thing and cutting it into the wood. And in that way I wouldn't feel embarrassed when we had lunch together."

"Yes, you said all of that. But you also said I didn't need a transplant. You said I already looked younger than you - even though I'm eight years older."

"Well, that's true. But I didn't for a minute think it would actually work. And I reckoned it would be a complete waste of money."

"But has it worked?"

"I think so. Now you do look younger than you did. It really is looking thicker."

Thicker. The magic word I'd longed to hear.

A little later, I start to wonder (again) just how thick the hair should be at this point. I don't want to bother

Mick with the *Before* and *After* pics, but I need some sort of benchmark. So I head back to the *Forum*, and there the mark is, thanks to Mark, who posted a blog in May, 2008.

Now, we don't have identical baldness problems, but Mark's transplant was carried out by Dr Farjo, almost exactly a year before me. 'Great,' I thought. 'I can compare notes.'

Mark, a professional musician, reveals he first considered a transplant back in 1997, and had consultations with three different surgeons.

'Two were hard sell operations, which put me off them. Then in 1998 I went to see Dr Bessam Farjo at their Harley Street clinic in London. He explained that this was the wrong time to begin surgery, as I may lose more hair, and it was too soon to accurately assess how much more hair I may lose.

The time was right, in Spring, 2007.

After 12 weeks I noticed new baby hairs coming through. By August friends were noticing my new hairs starting to show. By October my hair was starting to look good and I was no longer a shiny head. I felt like a farmer with a great harvest in front of him. It is now nearly twelve months since the transplant) and the results are still getting better. My self confidence is back Big Time.

Thanks, Mark. Now, this is August and here he is talking about getting a result by October. Suddenly, I feel uplifted.

The harvest news has worked.

'Your power is in your hair. What
a beautiful power it is.'

~ **Hedy Lamarr's** Delilah to Vic-
tor Mature's Samson.

27
Good Riddance to Bad Hair

EVEN though Mick has been saying since Day One that results don't really emerge until around Day One Hundred and Fifty, it's all too easy to push aside the comments of a professional. Sometimes you need the reassurance of an outsider. And Mark's blog offered that.

My new-found blithe confidence was certainly evident yesterday, August 15th. The Blonde took me along to her boss's barbeque and there I was looking around at other guys my own age and checking out their hairlines. And I realised that I had more hair that most.

Didn't they ever think about having some work done? No, I'm not being smug. (Okay, perhaps just a little). I just think that other bald men don't have to be, not when there is a relatively painless solution available. (Not with-standing the pain to the bank account.)

On the subject of pain, back in the office young Jonathan is asking how I got on at the dentist, if having a new crown fitted was close to Gestapo torture?

I replied that it wasn't.

"But it was stressful," Johnnie. "It's a white knuckle ride as soon as someone inserts a few knuckles and a whining object into your largest visible orifice."

"That's true," says my young Business Writer colleague.

"But it can't have been as painful as a transplant?"

"No, the transplant wasn't painful as it happens. There was a bit of discomfort for a few days, but the spray on antiseptic sorted that. And while I've heard of people who've died on a dentist's chair, no one has ever died from a hair transplant."

"How do you know, BB?"

"Good point, mate. I don't actually know. I'd better find out."

And it turns out someone *has* died during a hair replacement procedure, a Southern Californian, as recently as 2007.

'Walter Riley was 52 and went to Crown Cosmetic Surgery in Los Angeles a year ago for what he was told was a routine $4,000 hair transplant procedure,' reported the Los Angeles Examiner.

'The Riley family filed a malpractice a lawsuit and claimed an overdose of the anaesthetic lidocaine was to blame. '

I report my findings back to my work chum and, as expected he tosses the question at me; "Would you have thought twice about having a transplant if you'd known it could cause death?"

"No, I wouldn't Johnnie. It's a one-off instance. And if the death was caused, allegedly, by an anaesthetist's cock-up then I'd worry far more about going into hospital, where statistically there's a greater chance of something going wrong."

"Fair point."

"In any case, you could get killed driving to work in the morning, hurtling along at 70mph in a tin box with wheels. But we don't stop driving because of the road death stats. And in any case, the Riley death wasn't down to the actual transplant process, the surgery involved."

He takes my argument, chews on it, and seems satisfied. Then I take off to the canteen to see if the new tooth will allow me to chew on some toast. And I bump into page designer Mick, who asks how the hair is coming on.

Now, Mick is bald. Very bald. And he loves to crack jokes.

"I remember going to the doctor when I started to lose my hair," he says.

"I said 'Doctor have you got anything that can keep my hair in?' And he looked at me and said 'Here's a shoebox. Keep it in the loft'."

We laugh at the gag, but then I find myself slipping into my Mighty Hair Evangelist outfit.

"Don't you miss having hair, Mick? Would you want it back if you could have it?"

"No, not really. It doesn't bother me. When it began to go I just shaved it all off. And the wife quite likes it, so it's not a problem."

Mmm. I'm not convinced. And I take my toast and my inability to accept Mick's declaration back to the office. And I offer Mick's comment up to Jonathan and Barry. And I say I can't understand why someone with no hair could care less. And both look at me and grin.

Barry, in his late thirties, has zero hair on the top of his head, and Johnnie, just turned thirty, is fast receding. But what develops from the chat is something of a shocker.

Both are complimentary about my hair recovery, and hope I get a great result. And I believe them. However baldness, they maintain, doesn't bother them in the slightest.

"In fact, I'm glad not to have hair," says Barry, somewhat incredulously.

"What? I don't believe you for a minute."

"No, it's true. You see, I never had hair that I liked."

"Nonsense. Everyone likes having hair."

"You think? Well, mine was red for one thing. And always thin. And I used to have it pulled back in a ponytail to help make it look interesting.

"But it never worked. Then one day, when it became really thin I walked into a hairdressers' and asked for it to be shaved off. The hairdresser refused. She said blokes sometimes have their heads shaved and then regret it the following day. But I was adamant. I said it was time. And it was. And off it came. And you know I was glad. I didn't have to think about my hair ever again."

"Not quite, Barry. You've still got to shave it at the sides."

"Well, that's true. And it could do with a razor over it right now. But at least when I shave it, it takes a couple of minutes. And it costs nothing."

"Okay, you're happy enough to be bald. But, what if you could have your hair back, whether with a transplant or stem cell treatment. Would you go for it?"

"No, honestly. You see the point about my hair is that I never had hair I was particularly fond of. I don't lay awake at night thinking of my lost locks of lovely hair because they were never that in the first place."

Johnnie, young as he is, agrees with Barry.

"I never had great-looking hair either," he says of the thin covering that was once a tight, wiry curl.

"I never had a haircut or a style that I liked. I could never gel it or make it spiky or anything like that, the hair stuff that my pals did. There was nothing I could do with it. Every day was a bad hair day and even a set of ghds were never going to solve that problem.

"For me, going bald is not a major problem at all."

Well, my pal Jim had maintained it was never a problem. And now two of my work chums are saying the same thing. Can it be that some men can laugh in the face of a face without hair on top? Looking into my Hairfile I discover that top hairdresser Trevor Sorbie can.

'It never bothered me,' he maintained of his hair loss, 'except when I first started to go bald at the age of 24.'

And I found his comments hard to take, particularly from a man for whom hair is his working life.

But now I can understand why *some* don't need it. It suddenly dawns on me that there are blokes who don't need their hair. And that's because not everyone once had David Cassidy hair. Some were just once the wrong shade of ginger. Some had hair that was just too frizzy, hair that treated a comb with all the disdain the nit nurse once treated her charges. Some had hair that had once been the bane of their life.

Like Tommy McCafferty perhaps?

And I had the thought that if Tommy McCafferty had somehow, by some freak of nature had now lost his thick, red burst-cushion hair, perhaps he too would be happier to be hairless?

For the Mighty Hair Evangelist, this is a set-back. How can you help save the hair-losing men of the world if they don't want to be saved?

A couple of hours after the chat with Barry and

Jonathan however, I had another hair loss conversation, this time with Iain who runs the theatre across the road. (Now it has to be said I don't spend my days asking people about their personal experiences with baldness; those who know you've had a hair transplant like to comment.)

Iain told me he once was a drummer in a rock band. And at the age of 19, when Ozzy's Black Sabbath were in the charts with *Paranoid,* Iain's own Ozzy Ozbourne rock star waist-length hair suddenly disappeared into a black hole, the plug hole, never to be seen again.

At the time, Iain truly believed the capricious Hairgods were conspiring against him.

"I was in tears at the time," he says.

"I was a teenager and I needed my hair. I loved my hair. I thought I looked the bees knees. And when it went I cried for days, weeks afterwards. Of course, I had to go out and shave my head.

"But for me, losing my hair was the end of my youth, my wild teenage years. I actually felt suicidal, having this feeling that I wasn't young anymore.

"And of course you have to put up with the ribbing from your mates. How can you be a bald drummer in a rock n' roll band? And while it doesn't bother me now, in my fifties, I'd have given anything back then to have long hair again."

There. There is work out there for the Mighty Hair Evangelist. I just have to target those who don't have Tommy hair, and they're still at an age where they care.

I just thank God that my own hair didn't disappear so soon, like that of Iain and Sparky.

And at least I had time to watch the development of the transplant process - and hope that one day it would work.

'I am not the archetypal leading man. This is mainly for one reason: as you may have noticed, I have no hair.'

~ *Star Trek* star **Patrick Stewart**.

28
Growing Confidence

IT'S SATURDAY, August 23rd, and I'm off to play tennis in a couple of hours. But here's the thing. I haven't washed my hair. I reckon I'll be having a shower in about five hours time and I'll wash it then.

"So what?" I can hear you say. Well, here's what. It must be about ten years since I've hit the morning shower and not lathered my head with an expensive unguent.

It's a decade at least since I've dared to venture outdoors without having my hair thickened up with some full-bodied shampoo with some clever marketing name like *TresSemme Volume* or *Neutrogena* or *Bubblyhair* or whatever and then blow dried to add the air pockets that give a greater illusion of density.

Now, today, I feel bold enough not to have to do that. Okay, I'm not going to work, I'm going to a sweaty tennis centre where there will be very few people judging me, apart from thinking that I have the bucktoothed, ugly, spotty schoolboy of a backhand i.e. it leaves a lot to be desired.

But the point stands I'm feeling brave. The look in the mirror this morning made me feel happy. And (more) con-

fident. I'm no longer balding. I no longer have a Dracula
aversion to reflective glass. I'm the opposite of balding.
Whatever that is. Yes, I'm growing. But how much am I
growing? The only way I'll really know for sure if the hair
is thicker is if I get a positive comment from someone
who doesn't know I've had a transplant.

Yet, I know it's unlikely that a male will comment on
my hair, apropos nothing. Guys won't mention what's
going on with another guys head, unless it's something
they can be pleased about; i.e. something negative, like
growing hair loss (an oxymoron?) and you look like you've
holidayed in Alcatraz. In fact, the chances of blokes seeing an improvement on another man's head and making
a positive comment are as likely as Alcatraz re-opening.

Yesterday I attended a press conference and met up with
pal, Gavin (who has great hair) whom I haven't seen for a
few months.

"Hey, man, the hair looks great," he said.

"You've done the right thing."

And that was nice to hear. But it's not the comment I
wanted. I want/need to bump into someone who doesn't
know about the transplant who says to me 'Gosh, there's
something about you. There's a certain David Cassidy-
ness c1973. Could it be down to the fact you've got far
thicker hair?' Am I expecting too much? Yes. But deep inside my head I know there's an easy way to find out what's
really happening on top. I just have to work up the
courage to do it.

Meantime, encouragement comes at unexpected times
from unexpected places. Coming home from work I discover the Son of the Blonde, is back from the carefree
student life in Aberdeen to enjoy the even more carefree

life at home. But he has SkyPlused a programme for me. Now, that is unusual in itself. But he announces he has recorded the cop serial, *The Bill*. Which I don't watch.

"You will want to see it," he promises.

And you know, he is right. The episode features actor Shaun Williamson, whose early HT pics had prompted me to think about the procedure. Now, here he is on telly and his head looks fantastic.

Even SOB, with his thick-haired disinterested own head, is fascinated to see that a man with so little could now have so much.

"And you'll look better than he does," said SOB encouragingly.

"Why?"

"You don't have such a big head to cover. Well, not visually, anyway."

And I knew what he meant. And I was pleased. But not that pleased. This was an actor's head we were talking about. What about mine? I need to get a definitive judgement.

I have to talk to Mick. For the past few weeks the hair clinic manager has been suggesting I send him some new hair pics for comparison purposes. And today, September 4th, I did that. Our newspaper's ace photographer Martin took a new set of shots and I e-mailed them down to Manchester.

Now, I reckon, from looking in the mirror, that the hair result, so far looks ok. But what Mick did was dig out the original photos, the ones I had taken on the day of the transplant - before my head was shaved - and e-mail both the old and new back.

And as I open the file right now and look at the *Before*

shot I'm shocked. I had no idea I was so bald to begin with. I have virtually nothing on top. It's a stark reminder of the CCTV image I'd been frightened by in the garage. Incredibly, in the past few months I've somehow downloaded this image from my brain.

Perhaps I've managed to do this because I've become so used to having some hair on my head for the past month or so. But now I'm looking at the *After* photograph? Well, I'm astounded. It's absolutely incredible. I have to call Mick.

"Can you believe it, Mick? I can't!"

"It's looking good so far," says my hair man in Manchester with deliberate understatement.

"Remember, the new hair can continue to grow for up to a year. You're just four months into the process.

"But it's a very good start. And you're hair does seem to have grown exceptionally quickly."

"Quickly? The weeds in my garden don't grow as fast."

Okay, it's not back to the David Cassidy hair days, it's not even David Blane, but it's certainly not David Carradine in his *Kung Fu* days.

In such a short time there's a great covering. I'm taken aback. The careful, considered, cautious part of me had chosen to believe that the growing hair on my head was the returning hair. But now, here's the proof; I never had this much hair on the day of the HT.·

"Post the pics on the *Hair Forum*," says Mick. "Others will be interested to see how it's coming on."

He's right. And I do.

And I haven't yet got the racing bike with the Shimano 12 speed gears back but in my head I can see it being wrapped up for the Christmas post.

'President Kennedy had this great hair
and I read that somebody came and mas-
saged him because he had that back problem, but he would also get his hair pulled.
As men get older, the skin on their heads
tightens and the blood gets constricted.
Apparently, if you keep the skin loose
you're more apt to keep your hair.
So I just grab it with both hands and yank
on it while I'm watching the news.'

~ Acting veteran **Christopher Walken.**

29
Hair Blindness

IT'S almost the end of August and it's time to see Vinnie again. And I feel a little frisson of excitement because I want to show him my new hair. But he's busier than expected. It's a Friday night and he's had to squeeze in some bloke who wanted a last minute hair cut and Vinnie doesn't want to let him down because he gets him tickets for the Rangers games.

Well, what the hell. I'm looking forward to hearing Vinnie's comments.

Or I thought I would be.

The reality is quite different. He takes a quick look at my head before setting the razor to No 6 and says, "Yes, it's getting quite long on top. Just the spaces to be filled in."

"Spaces, Vinnie? It's still thin, sure. But what about the added thickness since last time? Are you off you're head, mate? Don't tell me the thought of free tickets to see Glasgow Rangers has fouled your free thought processes?"

Vinnie, not being psychic, doesn't hear my thoughts or register my dismay. And he proceeds to give me a cut faster than a keen ref's whistle for offside, buzzing it short at the sides but leaving the new top material untouched. I'd have thought a careful scissors blending in job would have been more appropriate, but Vinnie clearly doesn't agree. Or rather the part of his own head that should have weighed up that option is now sitting in the Govan Road stand.

But the rapid bzzzz isn't my big concern. It's the 'spaces' comment that's really tripped me up. There's only one thing for it. Another call to Mick. Luckily, I've got an excuse because I need to order up some more Finasteride; I really want to be doing everything I can to create new hair life. He promises to send it soon as. And he tells me not to worry about the thin hair, that it will thicken up.

What to do meantime, Mick? Is there anything I can do to encourage the process? What about laser combs? I'd heard about them but didn't realise that in 2007 they'd been approved by the American Food and Drug Administration.   After clinical trials running 26 weeks, the Hairmax Laser Comb was approved after it 'encouraged hair growth in males with androgenetic alopecia'.

Or bald blokes, as we know them.

"I'm not sure about the laser combs," says Mick. "I've seen the heads of a few people who've used them, but haven't seen a real improvement. Yet, one bloke I know swears he's had a result. It could be a placebo effect, it may work. I really don't know."

Can they do any harm?

"Only to your sense of self-esteem," he says, "if you expect great results and you don't get them." (And to your pocket. I've seen them advertised for over 300 quid.)

Should I give them a go? Maybe I'll get another comb for Christmas apart from the Stratton.

As is often the case, the chat with Mick wanders into interesting ground, the psychology of hair loss.

As a former sufferer, and having worked with hair loss clients for over ten years, Mick understands more than most the state of the hair-losing mind. And he offers up his reasons why other blokes won't want to acknowledge hair growth in another.

"Some men won't want to mention you've had a hair transplant because they'll feel they are intruding into your personal space. And some won't want to acknowledge you are looking better.

"But there are others who will know there's something different about you but can't quite put their finger on it."

Yes. Like those who failed to spot Sparky's wig.

Mick adds; "And, you have to remember this, some people won't bother to say positive things about your hair because they are too busy thinking about what they will doing that night or whatever.

"But don't worry. Your hair will be great.

"You'll be delighted."

I will. I will. I will.

If nothing else, willing it to grow should produce a result.

Mick's generosity of spirit when it comes to (some) men's reaction to bald men growing new hair however has a positive effect on me. I'm now a little more tolerant. I can smile at the knowing that when someone doesn't choose to acknowledge my growing hair it's not personal. It's a historical legacy. It's what men do. Attacks on those with less hair have always taken place. Baldness isn't just a condition, it's long been a device to show derision. As we know, Julius Caesar was forced into a combover, but it turns out he also came up with the laurel wreath decoration not to look imperious and god-like but to cover his overly-thin napper. The laurel wreath, it seems, was actually the ancient Roman equivalent of the baseball cap. And throughout history, many cultures have used hair removal as a form of humiliation, from Native American Indians to the French treatment of Nazi collaborators. The premise is that bald ness doesn't look good to the wider society. Sometimes, baldness is used as a form of servitude. Monks, for example. But monks don't get girlfriends.

David Cassidys get girlfriends. (And if you read his autobiography *Could It Be Forever*, you get the impression he had hundreds of thousands of them.) Ok, good-looking bald guys like Sean Connery get dates too. But it helps if they have a license to kill. (Although having been James Bond doesn't give you license to write anodyne autobiographies, evidenced by the news just in that Sir Shone has punted only 5,000 since the early August release.)

My pal Sparky certainly wouldn't disagree about how baldness can limit appeal. Teenage girls, as a rule, don't go for balding teenage boys. And he'd certainly agree with the contention that people prejudge the hairless as being 'weaker, less potent, less friendly, older and, in one study, less "good".'

A study carried out by the University of Michigan professor Daniel Moerman adds real weight to the argument. He asked college students to look at two drawings of the same man - one with hair and one without - and give their impressions.

196

'The data indicate the existence of a curious kind of prejudice in our society,' wrote Moerman.

'Across the board, the students thought that the bald subject was more intelligent, but considered the man with hair to be more attractive, more agreeable and younger.'

There's a thought that really does make me smile. While I was headed towards Barren Head Point people may have thought I was more intelligent than I am. But the correlation of that is with a (new) head of head I drop a few IQ points.

Will I now be regarded as a bubblehead because I have more hair? Well, that's not something that's likely to weigh heavily on my mind.

Instead, people may look at my crowning glory and think me more attractive and likeable.

And I can live with that.

30
Shorthand For Rubbish Hair

IT'S September 27th and five months after the transplant, and I'm developing a cosy relationship with my head. I'm quite happy to say hello in the mirror, although I don't linger quite as long as I did when I was 19.

But it's a pleasant exchange, and I can depart from my reflection with a warm feeling, a sense of well-being. This feeling is reinforced continually by pals. Last week I met Ford for lunch and his first comment, in spite of his business world being in a turmoil, was 'The hair looks f****** dynamite, by the way!'

Sure, some friends are slow to support the transformation process but that's okay. Out to dinner with a pal and his partner last week, my pal was asked by his what he thought of my new hair. He squinted in my direction and said; 'Looks alright.' And a few weeks ago I would have been upset that he couldn't have come up with a more colourful and supportive adjective. What the hell. Sometimes off-the-cuff comments are not what they're about. He may have been having a bad day.

That's the conclusion of my pal Steve. I'm telling him

about the danger in my judging people by their reaction to my head. "You will get a lot of negatives," he agrees. "What you've done is alter the balance in people's minds. They had a mental picture of you that was framed. They saw you a certain way and they have been comfortable with that. Now, what you've done is distort that picture. And it's no longer one they are comfortable with because it suited them to see you with no hair."

"Okay, but does that mean I can be comfortable with them? And, after all this is the age of equality. If women can be positive about someone else's improved appearance why can't men?

"Steve, if I can wear a new suit and get a compliment, why not a new head of hair?"

"Because the suit is an accessory," he says. "A temporary addition. The hair is you. What you've done is create a new you and it will be odd for some people to adjust to that.

"Give them time, mate. Give them a bit more time."

IT says a lot about your confidence when you can gleefully bang your head on a table.

This afternoon, October 8th, I'm in the lunchtime shorthand revision class and struggling. Badly. I can't seem to get it all down fast enough. And it's so frustrating I take to banging my head on the table. (Well, not actually banging, I'm really not that masochistic or tough.) But I do plop my head down hard(ish) in a rather theatrical display of despair. And it's a delightful moment. You see, back in March I would never have dropped my dome in front of eight others in the class, making my milk-white scalp entirely visible to the group. Now, subconsciously, six months later, I can do exactly that. Deep down I know that I now have enough up top.

While I may struggle to write the 80 wpm shorthand for 'transplant surgery' or indeed 'dihydrotestosterone' I can at least flop my new head of hair onto whichever hard, low-level public table I choose with a complete lack of self-awareness.

Delightfully, those around aren't focused on my foliicly-challenged head.

They are simply thinking 'The man's an idiot.'

And that's great. It's awesome. I now have hair. How much? Well, I've got a frontal hairline now, of sorts. And that means the 'baldy' jokes will stop. Why? They'll be in-appropriate. To be classed as 'bald' requires a head as shiny as a newly-frozen ice rink. And people won't see that when they look at me. Hair experts point out that when you meet someone they first focus on the area immedi-ately above the eyes. They see the hairline. They don't see the top of your scalp - unless you're a snooker player or a very small person or they're looking at you from the top of a bus.

You see, if you have some hair, then the worst name you can be called is 'balding' or 'thinning'. And people (i.e blokes) who want a laugh at your expense are extremely unlikely to call you a 'thinning bastard!'

Could my hair be described right now as 'thinning'? Yes, it could be if those attaching the label didn't know the reality, that it's actually thickening.

But already I'm building up hope there's more to come.

'When I was in college theatre I played a
65 year-old man and as I shaved my
head, to get the Male Pattern Baldness
effect. But then I used greasepaint
rather than powderto cover up my hairline and it destroyed my follicles.
It was a traumatic experience.
It was a train wreck of a situation and I
wore hair pieces as a young actor.
But you know, the baldness has shaped
my career. And I'm glad that it has.'

~ *The Shield's* Vic Mackey, actor
Michael Chiklis.

31
Obama's Great Hairday

IT'S now seven months PT. The international credit crunch has kicked in and the financial world and the structures of commerce are collapsing like a Sixties bee-hive in a thunderstorm. And, if nothing else, it confirms that baldness and intelligence don't go hand in hand.

Many of the world's top-level bankers have receding hair, yet they've led us blindly into world recession. Mind you, the bankers and brokers have paid themselves some very decent bonuses over the years. So perhaps they're not so stupid after all. We can only hope that their bonuses have been spent on property portfolios that are now worthless and there's nothing left in the pot for hair work.

All the newspaper talk of recession however has meant that a new baldness breakthrough didn't get the column inches it would otherwise have collected. Scientists reported they 'have found a cause for male-pattern baldness - the hair loss gene.'

As is the way with most discoveries, the identification of Chromosome 20 came about as a by-product of another experiment, in this case it was in heart and artery disease. 'So, as a lark, we decided we would try to find the genes that increase people's susceptibility to male-pattern baldness,' said Dr. Brent Richards, an assistant professor in the departments of medicine and human genetics at McGill University in Toronto.'

I had to laugh at the comment. A lark? Millions of desperate men await a cure for baldness. The money spent on hair transplantation alone in the United States was more than $115 million in 2007, according to news reports. And global revenues for medical therapy for male-pattern baldness recently surpassed $405 million.

Regardless, the gene discovery is good news, with the implication being that having found the gene, it can then be switched off, or adjusted.

Well, for the next generation, perhaps.

'It will be a long time before the discovery will bear any fruit,' said Dr Richards of Chromosome 20.

'But it does definitely expand our understanding of what seems to influence male-pattern baldness.'

Now, there was a time when that story would have left me feeling both excited and disappointed. So close and yet . . .

However, my new, growing hair makes my hair bi-polarity redundant. I can smile knowing I have enough not only to be able to show scalp but to make a difference to my appearance.

Out for a walk at lunchtime I bump into Linda, a workmate who jumped ship a year ago to become freelance.

"You're looking great," says my perennially upbeat pal.

"But there's something different about you."

"Linda, you're an angel."

"Why? What is it? And there *is* something different about you."

"Well, it could be the hair."

"Why? Have you just had it cut?"

"No. I've had a hair transplant."

"You have not! It just looks as though you've got a new hair style."

"No, I haven't got a new hair style. (Not since Vinnie took off on holiday to hurricane-blown Houston.) And if you remember, by the time you left the paper I didn't have much to cut. In fact it was almost sides only."

"Well, it looks fantastic. You look so different."

I feel my head is headed in the right direction. And there isn't a day goes by now without someone in the office mentioning the improvement. What I am noticing however, is a lot more hairs in the plug hole after the morning shower. Is this because there is so much more on my head? Am I losing some of the new hair already? I have to remind myself that up to 100 hairs are lost every day anyway. And the new ones are pushing their way up onto my head as we speak.

BET you Lewis Hamilton is wishing he had a few new hairs about to appear on his head.

I'm watching television, it's November 2nd, and the boy racer has just won the Formula 1 World Championships. And I'm thinking he may now be worth around £150m but he could do with spending a few quid on new hair. Lewis's dad is bald. And at just 23 years-old Lewis is motoring fast in exactly the same direction.

Mind you, his Pussycat Doll girlfriend doesn't seem to have noticed his departing hairline at all. And there's no doubt the fastest man in the world can afford to pit stop any time he likes at any one of the world's very best hair treatment centres. But another Hamilton thought enters my head. He's a little unlucky in the hair department. Black men are four times less likely to lose their hair as white men. (Statistics show that Russian men have the strongest hair.)

A couple of days later however, the stat relating to black men comes to mind again. Barack Obama has not only won out against DHT and anything else that can contribute to baldness, he's just become the first black US president. But all the signs are he'd never have made it if he'd been bald. Even though he was up against an old reactionary and a deer shooter who can't remember which newspapers she reads, if he'd not had good hair he wouldn't have made it past the Primaries.

How do I know this to be true? Well, Americans, as a race, don't elect bald men. The U.S. has had more than five bald Presidents, but Americans haven't voted one into office in 52 years, since Dwight Eisenhower. And he beat another baldy, Adlai Stevenson. And that was in 1956, when 20th Century Fox released *The King and* I, starring Yul Brynner as the King of Siam, when baldness, for a short period, a very short period, had some cachet.

Recently *Men's Health* magazine's style and grooming editor Sarah Cremer, claimed that for the majority of men a full head of hair is still inextricably bound up with the idea of 'youth, virility and ultimately attractiveness'. And she's right. She adds however; 'It's ironic really that most surveys show that women don't care if men are balding.

'Much more likely to be a turn-off is the scrape-over, the spray-on hair in an aerosol, the badly fitting toupee, or even worse - an awful, self-conscious obsession with hair loss.'

And she may be right on that too, but I'm not quite so

sure. Give women the choice and I'd argue they'd go for the man with the David Cassidy hair every time.

And that thought makes me wonder. I wonder how the Hairgod himself is getting on as far as David Cassidy hair goes?

Has he managed to hold onto it?

The only thing to do is ask him.

'I'm a man and I will beat up
anybody who tries to tell me that I am
not a man just
because my hair is thinning.'

~ **Bruce Willis.**

32
Hairgod Support

IT'S Friday night, 6pm, and I'm ready to leap into the weekend. But first there is one more phone interview to do. Now, normally I wouldn't hang around on a Friday night to chat to a celeb. Who's that important they can't wait 'till Monday? But this evening the subject is a bit special. It's the Hairgod himself.

Yes, David Cassidy.

The star is back in town with a concert special and I'm to interview him for the newspaper. And is always the case with Cassidy, he gives great conversation. He's open and honest. But here's the thought; will he talk about hair and any possible hairloss?

I've Googled him 'till I'm blue in the face and can't find an interview where he's spoken on the subject.

What the hell, after 45 minutes or so of talking about his life and family - and getting a nice exclusive - I throw the hair thought at him.

"David, I've just had a hair transplant. And I'm writing a book about it. And one of the themes in the book is I want to regain the David Cassidy hair I once had as a teenager."

"Me too!" he says laughing.

"Okay, here's the question. I've been looking at some photographs over the years David, and I'm guessing here, and I may be wrong, but it looks as though you've had a few follicles inserted. Is it the case?"

There's a pause, and then a slight laugh from the Hairgod.

"You know, no one has ever asked me about this. But yes. Back in 1990 I once had a part in a little movie made by Francis Ford Coppola's company called *Spirit of '76*, about time travellers.

"And Coppola wanted me to have the '76 hairstyle. And so I grew it out, and it looked pretty much like it once did. But I noticed that it wasn't *quite* the same."

The Hairgod turned time traveller had been affected by the ravages of time.

And the evil DHT.

"I was missing part of my hair line. And the back was a bit thin. And I thought 'Jesus!' So I figured 'I'll go in and have it fixed.' And I did."

David took himself off to one of the best transplant surgeons in the States.

"And they put 60 grafts in my hair, these micrografts. And it was friggin' painful. Unfortunately, I have a very sensitive scalp and a really low threshold for it. And I suffered.

"But I went through with it."

And again, one more time.

"Then I said to myself that next time I'd really go through with it. So I went back and said to give me the maximum amount of grafts they could, but the most they would do is 200 grafts.

"Of course, nowadays they do around 2,000."

"Well, in my case, 3200, David."

"Wow!

Regardless, David got a very good result from his 260-odd grafts from his two procedures.

"My hair is good enough," he says.

"You know, I wish I'd waited and had that amount done at the one time. But you know what, it's fine. I've got enough and I don't think too much of it is falling out."

He adds, grinning; "We don't have the volume we used to have. But that was 18 years ago and I'm not going back to do it (a transplant) again. I'm letting it go, baby."

By 'letting it go' he means he's not worrying about it. His hair is in good shape although I'm not so sure about the way he styles it these days. It's swept back, all very tidy but rather corporate, a little too much Eighties/Gordon Gekko.

Nonetheless, David Cassidy still has very good hair, particularly for a 58 year-old. And while he no longer has his fringe that doesn't mean I have to give up the goal of having one by Christmas.

"David, I'm going to get as close to David Cassidy hair as I can by the end of this hair trip. It's my dream."

"I hope you do, buddy. And you need to get me the photographs of your hair when you grow it out.

"I need to see how it turns out."

And you will, David. Just as soon as that DC fringe kicks in.

'There's nothing more contemptible than
a bald man who pretends to have hair.'

~ Latin poet **Martial** (Marcus Valerius
Martialis)

33
Comb For Christmas?

WE'RE now at the beginning of December, eight months since Dr Farjo and the team brought new follicular life to my scalp. And the result is really great.

The fringe is back, that glorious neat, dark curtain of hair that has been absent for the best (or rather the worst) part of twenty years.

Now, my overly thick eyebrows don't look quite so Brezhnev. And while I still don't have the thickness of hair I once had, the volume is increasing.

Mick reminds me it can take up to a year before all the new hair emerges so by the time Spring comes around many more follicles will have sprung up. Fantastic.

I'm still touching my head quite a lot; taking quiet comfort from feeling the little spikes of new hair - but not religiously.

However I'm still a bit OCD when it comes to noticing other men's hairlines. While most Manchester United supporters have been worrying about Wayne Rooney's recent inability to hit the back of the net, I've been worrying about his hair loss. (Perhaps it's no real surprise he hasn't scored since he shaved what was left of his balding head; Samson's goal strength gone?) And it was concerning, but not surprising, to hear that he's been getting a hard time in the dressing room over his lost hair.

That's what men do to the balding.

What the soccer star can't do, it seems, is to undergo baldness treatment. Aside from the fact he's probably too young to have a transplant (his donor area is still receding) chances are his team-mates would line up to take shots at him.

Still, perhaps when the Mighty Hair Evangelist helps spread the word the highly judgmental young footballers who earn 120k a week and often add to that with endorsements for slick hair grooming products may think twice about ribbing the hairless.

Maybe.

It's not just footballers however who could do with lightening up on the critical hair improvement front. Journalists are every bit as culpable. Like John Naish of the *Sunday Times*. Just recently he wrote of actor John Cleese; 'The Python star has gone from comedy icon to laughing stock with the ultimate sad op: he said this week (on *Richard and Judy's* TV show) he'd just had a transplant. "I have got this very strange skull, very pointy, and I don't like wearing wigs."

'Oddly, this doesn't seem to be the first time Cleese, 69, has had a cover-up: In 1989 he revealed he had undergone a transplant and joked: "I redistributed my hair on socialist principles".'

The *Sunday Times* writer however wasn't laughing with Cleese when it came to the actor's twin attempts at self-improvement.

'Is this a double dose of vanity John?' he wrote. 'Or are we just splitting hairs?' Miaow! This is the reason why actors (and normal people) are reluctant to admit to having hair work done, why people like JC bare their soul and end up having to wear a hair shirt.

I take it you've got hair Mr Naish? I haven't seen a picture byline, but I'll be looking out for one.

Meantime, I'll be getting a new byline pic taken for my own paper. It's an incredible feeling, to get a foto taken in which I'll actually look better than the last one I had done about five years ago.

Of course, most people won't notice the change. They don't. Unlike in olden days, the dolls hair days when you could spot a hair transplant from a hundred yards, no one has been able to tell that I've had hair transferred.

It's fantastic.

But not entirely.

My new hair transformation doesn't register with most people. They make a comment that there's something different about me, but they're not sure what it is. It's because the transformation has been gradual. If I'd gone from being completely bald ie. no hair on my head whatsoever, and suddenly had the amount I have now, it would attract attention.

But I've gone from having an almost bald crown - with hair at the sides - to having a decent amount of hair on the crown - with hair at the sides - over a period of months. It's not that dramatic a leap – to other people.

And while there's a part of me who wants someone to say, 'God, you got so much more hair than you had before. How come?' I know that's not what happens.

For example, last Friday night in the pub one of the Blonde's pals, who knew nothing of the transplant, looked at me and said 'There's something different about you.'

'Yes? What?'

'I don't know. It's your face.'

'Same face, Val.'

'No, it's not. It seems, well, I don't know what it is, but it seems softer.'

'Could it be the hair?'

'Yes, maybe. Have you changed your hairstyle or something?'

'Well, actually . . .'

Okay, Val may never make a detective, but then again she's fairly typical. Those who aren't close don't readily absorb the difference.

But the main thing is *I* notice the difference.

* * * * * * * * * * * * *

MANKIND doesn't need hair of course, with the exception of the dust-catching hairs in our ears and nose and our eyelashes and eyebrows. It's not that cold anymore.

But on the other hand we really need hair, especially when we're young, because society still equates hair with youth.

You need hair to be able to gel it, make it stick up/out, to dye it blond/pink/blue and shock your dad senseless.

You need hair if only to show you don't need hair, so that you can shave it off in a fit of pique, moment of madness/ need to get rid of the head lice you picked up in the cheap youth hostel in Kuala Lumpar.

And you need hair to attract the opposite sex. Or even the same sex.

Hair, you see, is not just a feature, a clump of keratin, it's a statement, a declaration.

Yes, as you get older you don't need as much hair,

thanks to the fact most people around you are facing the same loss. And there's a greater chance you'll have a partner, so there's less need to peacock yourself. (Sure, you can wear funky specs or wear hats or loud shirts but that's all a bit Jim Carrey).

But there's still a desire. There's still a yearn to use a comb, maybe dab on a little Brylcreem like your dad once did.   There's still a notion to try out a new hairstyle – comb it backwards, comb it forwards, make it stick up at the front, just a little, because there's a little of the Rod Stewart in all of us.

And that's not just his legions of exes talking.

Yet, what's really fantastic about having hair is that it allows for a series of wonderful *Nos* to be grafted onto your life.

No more suncream on the scalp.

No more big hats.

No fear of bending down.

No more wincing at bald jokes.

No more patronising hairdressers.

No longer having to rush past mirrors.

No more attempts at self-delusion that you really have a decent covering of hair but you're about as convincing as Demi Moore in *Strip Tease*.

There are more *Nos*.

No more patting your few hairs into place when you step out of the lift in the morning.

No fear of plugholes.

No fear of passport photographs.

No fear for others close to you, (like your mum) who you know has been worried that you're worried about your ever-increasing hair loss.

Now, some may say if I had a big enough personality in the first place I'd have been able to play down the hair loss, that if I were a fully rounded human being I'd be happy as I were.

And perhaps that's true. But I'm not. I'd be happier to be 17 again. Hair-wise that is.

Now, I'll most likely never achieve that. I haven't got my David Cassidy c1973 hair back.

Yet, my life is now looking more like a Frank Capra movie by the minute.

I can see the snow outside and the log fire indoors. And I can see my Christmas stocking hanging over the mantelpiece.

And you know what, I bet there's a nice Stratton comb inside.

The End

All I Want For Christmas Is A Comb

By Ian Pattison.

ALL I want for Christmas is a comb
and follicles soft and lush across my dome
spread carelessly like hay on rich red loam
or surfers riding waves of ocean foam.
Yes, all I want for Christmas is a comb.

How fondly I still see combs of yesteryear
I scent their Brillcremed tang and shed a tear
the xylophone thrum I once strummed with my thumb
would send puffs of jolly dandruff in the air
like indoor snow on a day of festive cheer
Now all I want for Christmas is a comb!

If you think me vain then please do understand
my baldness was not worked by my own hand
free will had I none, the deed was naturally done
for my body would stay white as my head grew tanned
the angels razed my fuzz at God's command
and left me praying to my maker for a comb!

Now man is mortal, that much is clearly understand, (stood)
we see the trees and only later see the wood,
the path grows dark, the day winds down the hill
all must part who may be friends and lovers still.
But the bald man's loss is much more harshly dealt
for parting with a parting is twice felt
thus he is doubly damned and lost and far from home
Yet all he asks for Christmas is a comb!

Mine, of course, is not an ode to hair
for we cannot praise that which is not there
The plough may furrow, the reaper reap
the barber bag our hair to keep
our helpless heads grow shiny as we sleep...

And hence the poignant nature of this pome,
Oh, all I want for Christmas is a comb.
all year long this mantra I'll intone -
All I want for Christmas is a comb!